EVERYWOMAN'S GUIDE

# EVERYWOMAN'S GUIDE TO NATURAL HEALTH

*by*

CAPTAIN GEOFFREY T. WHITEHOUSE
D.S.C., F.R.S.H., M.N.I.M.H.

THORSONS PUBLISHERS LIMITED
Wellingborough, Northamptonshire

First published 1974

ISBN 0 7225 0277 X

Typeset by Specialised Offset Services Ltd., Liverpool
and printed and bound by
Whitstable Litho Limited, Whitstable, Kent.

# CONTENTS

# INTRODUCTION

Judging by the ever-increasing volume of correspondence which reaches me daily from women and girls concerning gynaecological problems, it has become more and more obvious that publication of a comprehensive book on the natural health approach to women's ailments should be delayed no longer.

Hence this book, a number of chapters of which are based upon my articles which have appeared in *Here's Health*, and I am grateful to the publishers of this magazine for giving me permission to do this.

The central theme in all my writing on women's ailments is that we, the unorthodox, whether we be medical herbalists, homoeopaths or naturopaths, have much of value to offer to women who have a dislike of surgical operations on the one hand, and of the menace to their well-being arising out of over-dependence on potent drugs on the other. A realistic and well-tested alternative is usually available.

Readers of the book will find as they pass from one chapter to another that reference to various gynaecological ailments; to appropriate treatment for these; to the problems of teenage girls in what we have come to regard as the era of 'permissiveness'; to the contraceptive pill and to hormone imbalance and its significance, tend to become repetitive. My excuse for this, if any is needed, is that there is a consistency in what I have to say about all these matters and it is hoped that repetition will serve the purpose of driving home the points I wish to make in the minds of my readers.

At no time have I sought to unreservedly criticize or denigrate our contemporaries in the medical profession, the great majority of whom are just as dedicated in their desire to heal and reduce suffering as we are. I firmly believe, however, that our approach to the amelioration of ill-health is in many ways more logical and more practical than that of the generality of physicians and surgeons.

One of the greatest disadvantages from which the medical profession suffers in dealing with illness is the lack of co-operation between the many branches of medicine itself and

between physicians and surgeons. Although our medical contemporaries are just as much aware as we are that common
sense demands that the whole person be treated and not merely
the symptoms presented, this principle is usually ignored in
practice.

The most common major operation to which women have to
submit is that of hysterectomy. Sometimes, but by no means
always, we can agree that the operation is unavoidable, but I
know of few cases in which there has been co-operation
between surgeon and physician to ensure that the ability of the
patient to undergo the operation with a minimum of distress
and make a rapid recovery subsequently is given the consideration it ought to have.

There is clearly a strong case here for building up the
patient's general health and healing capacity through good
nutrition supported, if necessary, by supplementary nutrients
derived from natural sources. Over and over again I have seen
the value of this precaution demonstrated by patients in my
care.

Another bone of contention lies in disregard by the medical
profession of the principle that in treating disease we must seek
and eradicate the cause and not deal solely with the symptoms
presented. The average doctor is sensible enough to realize that
this is a thoroughly sound principle but there are very few who
adhere to it.

Perhaps it will be thought cynical if I say that, since without
surgery there would be no need of surgeons, the latter are apt to
justify their existence by advocating surgery when less drastic
measures would suffice. Criticism must be levelled at the
opinion commonly expressed by gynaecologists, who are also
surgeons, that once a woman has passed her childbearing age her
womb has become a useless and redundant organ and is best
removed if it gives any trouble. In the aggregate, millions of
women have been ruthlessly deprived of this organ as though it
is of no consequence. In some cases there is no adverse reaction
but my correspondence indicates beyond possible doubt that in
many more cases the result is disastrous from both the mental
and physical angle. Sensitive women will suffer a deep sense of
feminine deprivation and severe depression, whilst in many
others the menopausal disorders they have to endure, perhaps
for years, are far worse than would have been the case if their
menopause had been a natural one.

It would seem that the management of pregnancy is a service hardly recognized by doctors and yet it is of the utmost importance, for the sake not only of the mother-to-be, but also of the child she will bear. In our profession most of us will take exceptional care of our patients when they become pregnant, with emphasis on sound and wholesome nutrition and physical aid through manipulative treatment and the teaching of exercises. Results are in most cases gratifying in the extreme with easy delivery, and rapid recovery, and the reward of an offspring sound in constitution and happy and contented in disposition.

Among the products of the pharmaceutical industry to which strong objection must be taken is the contraceptive pill, which must surely be their supreme bonanza. It is very popular with doctors because it represents an easy way of prescribing hormone treatment. Its use is not confined by any means to the purpose for which it was originally intended. Nowadays doctors prescribe it for a variety of gynaecological disorders associated with menstruation. I have repeatedly condemned the pill because of the virtual certainty that its effect on many women could be gravely detrimental to their health, both general and gynaecological, especially in the long run. I particularly object to the administration of the pill to teenage girls who have the misfortune to suffer from menstrual failure. The long-term effect on the welfare of their reproductive organs, so intricate physically and so delicately balanced physiologically, could be disastrous. Medical herbalists provide many safe remedies for the treatment of this disorder. As for contraception, my advice to women is to continue to rely on the older and well-tested methods which, if properly used, are safe and harmless. A full discussion of the case against the pill will be found in Chapter Twenty-One.

As I have already said, complaints against the medical profession must be tempered by an acknowledgement that the majority of doctors do their best to ease the sufferings of mankind within the limitations imposed upon them. A growing number of doctors are coming over to our way of thinking and the number is certain to increase in the course of time. Unfortunately, whilst the General Medical Council permits a doctor to 'call in' an unorthodox practitioner if he wishes to, there is no reciprocity. A medical doctor is forbidden by his Council to co-operate with the unorthodox practitioner in any way. He cannot divulge case histories to them, even if asked to do so by a patient, or co-operate in other respects. We cannot obtain case-histories of our patients from hospitals they have previously attended. Because of this unfortunate barrier it is the patient who suffers the greatest disadvantage, to say nothing of her disgust about having to subscribe heavily to the National Health Service which has failed to restore her health, and then having to pay once again to cover the fees and remedies of the unorthodox practitioner to whom, in desperation, she has been obliged to turn.

Fortunately, the barrier is giving way and I, myself, have received useful co-operation from several doctors in recent years. With the coming into force of the Medicines Act of 1968, medical herbalism is now legally recognized. This important milestone is likely to have far-reaching results in due course. Whilst the Bill was being debated before its enactment a gratifying number of Members of Parliament, including some who are doctors, came out in support of medical herbalism. To Mrs Joyce Butler M.P. belongs most of the credit, for her efforts in Parliament have resulted in the Medicines Act recognizing and favouring at least one section of unorthodox medicine, and we are exceedingly grateful to her.

My acknowledgement is due to hundreds of women dwelling in all parts of the U.K., in Eire and in each of the five continents who have, during the past fourteen years, sought my assistance in finding solutions for their health problems and private dilemmas of various kinds. They are of all ages and all nations. They have caused me to study unceasingly and ponder deeply in seeking the right solutions, and are thus entitled to much of the credit for the appearance of this book, and for the helpfulness to other women of its contents.

## 1

# NATUROPATHIC GYNAECOLOGY

In the minds of many who have occasion to dwell upon the matter, the gynaecologist will be associated with surgical operations. Common among these are hysterectomies, ovariectomies, salpingectomies, cauterization of the cervix, the 'scrape' and removal of 'the lot' One cannot, as a naturopath, practise exclusively among women without learning a great deal about procedures on the other side of the fence.

A surprising number of hospital nurses desert the orthodox in favour of the more conservative school when they themselves need help, because they have become disillusioned by the readiness with which the surgical removal of organs of reproduction is carried out. They are appalled by the ever-increasing number of young women who are admitted to hospital with gynaecological disorders, only to find that the sole remedy available is recourse to surgery. Hysterectomies performed upon women still in their twenties are not uncommon, whilst women who have passed the menopause are often urged to submit to this operation, whether necessary or not, on the grounds that the womb has become a redundant organ anyway. Many women strongly object to this attitude.

Although this undue readiness among orthodox gynaecologists to resort to hysterectomy is all-too-common, I should not like it to be thought that there are no exceptions. I am well aware that some of the most eminent gynaecologists are also the most considerate. When confronted with a non-malignant uterine tumour, commonly known as fibroid, they will take infinite pains to remove it without inflicting irreparable damage on the uterus itself. I have known cases in which multiple tumours totalling in volume that of a six-month pregnancy have been successfully excised, leaving the uterus virtually intact. Such consideration is not necessarily confined to women of childbearing age but is also accorded to older patients. Happily, not all gynaecologists regard the post-menopausal womb as a redundant organ.

## Serious Shortcomings
That the work of these good men, nevertheless, has serious

shortcomings is no fault of theirs but of the system of which they are a part. The orthodox medical profession is organized in such a way that it is not possible for a gynaecologist, or any other specialist for that matter, to follow the golden rule of Nature Cure by treating the whole person. The orthodox gynaecologist is not concerned with the preparation of his patient for the ordeal of an operation, nor with her after-care. On occasion the woman's panel doctor will give advice on this important aspect of her general welfare but more often than not she is left entirely to her own devices.

It would be incorrect to give the impression that gynae-cologists are totally unconcerned with gynaecological problems that do not involve surgery. Nevertheless, it is by reason of their skill as surgeons that they are most likely to gain distinction.

The treatment of such disorders as dysmenorrhoea, menstrual failure, leucorrhoea, and vaginal pruritus are more often dealt with by general practitioners, with an impressive variety of drugs which have been brought to their notice by the persistent publicity of the pharmaceutical industry, rather than by gynaecologists. The contraceptive pill, because of its hormone content, is a prime favourite.

In cases of infertility, testing the potency of the fallopian tubes would be within the sphere of the gynaecologist and so would the extremely delicate but seldom successful surgical operation of unblocking tubes which are structurally defective.

Readers are likely to be thinking that it is all very well to criticize our gynaecologists but what alternative do we have? I am afraid the answer is not encouraging because what we might describe as the bloodless gynaecologist, or more precisely, the naturopathic gynaecologist, is hard to find.

Before the hospitals were nationalized under our National Health system, a naturopath had no difficulty in attaching himself to a gynaecologist as a student, thereby gaining all the experience he required through attending during the examin-ation of the patients and at operations.

If women are to continue to have an alternative to the kind of orthodox gynaecology which I have described, there is an urgent need for those of us who have enjoyed facilities to acquire knowledge no longer available, to pass on our know-ledge to a new generation of naturopaths and medical herbalists. This could be done in the few teaching establishments we have if practitioners were prepared to give up their practices for this purpose, but it seems they are not. An alternative would be to revive the ancient system, long defunct, which gave us the apothecaries' apprentice.

I feel sure my readers, of whom so many are keenly interested in the alleviation of women's problems, would like to know what my views are about the training of the kind of gynaecologist we are discussing.

Whether the student be man or woman, when it comes to suitability for the calling it is very much a matter of temperament. Some among us are insensitive and down-to-earth, whilst others are filled with compassion for the suffering of others and prepared to dedicate themselves to its alleviation. When dedication dictates our actions in this sphere of the healing art there is a double gain. We, ourselves, derive endless satisfaction from our efforts whilst the object of our administrations is far more likely to benefit.

I would not myself undertake to train a student as a naturopathic gynaecologist who did not have the right temperament. Given this the task might not be difficult.

From this point onwards when using the term gynaecologist, I shall be referring to the ideal I should try to build up in the mind of a student.


## Miracle of Reproduction

First of all, we must never lose sight of the fact that as the female counterpart of genus man, which we accept as the highest form of life, woman is the supreme example of the miracle of reproduction. For this reason alone we must venerate her.

A basic fact to bear in mind is that woman is far more complex, not only physically but also mentally, than man. The present-day tendency to disregard this difference is not ultimately favourable to women and should be strongly resisted.

We must have a deep and ever-ready sympathy for women who seek assistance in alleviating their ailments or solving their private problems. One is amply rewarded for the time taken in sorting out emotional problems by the gratitude so often, and sometimes so movingly, expressed. The therapeutic value of these talks about problems of a profoundly personal nature cannot be over-estimated.

To be worthy of his salt a gynaecologist must also be a psychologist, whilst an extensive knowledge of sexual customs and problems was never so essential as it is today. In my view, a gynaecologist must also be a sexologist since so many of the disorders to which women are prone are due to sexual causes.

Among the disorders the naturopathic gynaecologist will be called upon to treat are menstrual failure and irregularities; lack of tone, underdevelopment and displacement of the womb; uterine fibroids, ovarian cysts and tumours, leucorrhoea, infertility, difficulties in intercourse and change of life ailments. More general disorders to which women are prone are varicose veins, intestinal complaints, nervousness and insomnia.

Foremost in mind will be the principle that the *whole person* must be considered and not merely the symptoms that are presented.

Treatments regularly employed in Nature Cure are controlled fasting and attention to diet, nutrition, and hydrotherapy — which embraces the judicious use of hot and cold water to promote circulation and the eliminative processes. Patients are encouraged to live sensibly and wholesomely, taking proper care of their bodies. Natural healing processes are aided by the prescription, when necessary, of herbal or homoeopathic remedies.

In many gynaecological ailments it will be found that what we regard as pure Nature Cure, wherein no medicines of any kind are administered, will not succeed. The well-being of the patient must at all times be our main consideration and this in my view justifies the employment of safe remedies which have stood the test of centuries of time and are thus a very different proposition from many of today's drugs, of which we are so suspicious. To give a few examples; in my experience such disorders as uterine fibroids, ovarian cysts, leucorrhoea, pruritus and non-malignant mastitis cannot be kept under control, let alone cured without the employment of our type of medication.

The management of pregnancy is a sphere in which the naturopathic gynaecologist, with the necessary training and experience, can achieve exceptionally gratifying results. Having been trained to treat the *whole person* there is no greater asset than this, where the welfare of a pregnant woman and the baby she will bear are concerned.

## Infertility

Infertility can be due to so many causes that its treatment offers great scope for the resourcefulness of the practitioner. Wives or couples who come to us for treatment vary greatly in their experience. In some cases no previous treatment, orthodox or otherwise, has been given, whilst in others the whole gamut of treatments, as laid down in the textbooks, have been tried without success. It is then that Nature Cure, with its entirely different approach to the problem, is resorted to in desperation.

In my experience the aspects of infertility most often neglected are the psychological, the nutritional and the physiological. In point of fact, the latter approach, involving manipulative treatment and the teaching of specially designed exercises, holds great promise.

Research into nutritional problems has shown that when infertility is due to hormone deficiency, as is frequently the case, the deficiency can often be made good by the prescription of an appropriate combination of naturally derived vitamins. If, at the same time, herbal precursors and homoeopathic remedies designed to unlock and activate the vital forces of the body are administered, a natural sequence of events can be set in motion with very promising prospects.

In the marital sphere there is much scope for the sympathetic and experienced gynaecologist. It may surprise readers to learn how many women there are who, although married — maybe for months or years — have not been successful in consummating their marriage. With skill on the part of the practitioner, resulting from experience and the exercise of patience, this difficulty can almost always be overcome.

It has become particularly desirable, now that the pill appears to have been accepted by the medical profession as the contraceptive of first choice, that women who are rightly alarmed at this further example of the all-too-ready use of drugs, and who greatly fear the possible consequences, should have an alternative means of obtaining protection. This the naturopathic gynaecologist can provide.

The world of today is full of perplexity for teenagers of both sexes but for the young girl, who is so much more vulnerable, the difficulties that arise can be particularly devastating.

Powerful influences such as the cinema, the television, the popular press and, most of all, subtle advertising directed at the impressionable minds of the young, all too often cause them to drift away from the steadying influence of their parents. Others again may be the products of a broken home. The results of these trends are often seen by me when young girls come along for advice or treatment, either by themselves or with a parent or a girl or boy friend. They are always received with sympathy and understanding and their needs are attended to with the seriousness and delicacy they warrant. Among disorders, the most common in young girls concerns menstruation, which can be either painful or erratic or non-existent. Other girls come because they are doubtful about the normality of their physical development and proportions and may suspect 'glandular' trouble. They may be too fat or too thin or too boyish or underdeveloped, or their 'vital statistics' do not agree with what they have read. Some need little more than reassurance and advice whilst others need treatment of some kind or other.

In a surprising number of cases appointments are made by their parents for young girls to be given talks on the 'facts of life' because they themselves are reluctant to do so and are not happy about the manner in which this important subject is dealt with in schools.

### Importance of Periodical 'Check-up'

I place a great emphasis on the importance to women of the periodical 'check-up'. The majority of ailments to which women are prone, including malignancy, could be prevented from developing if suspicious conditions were detected in good time. Unhealthy conditions are carefully noted in the course of an examination and steps are then taken to provide treatment designed to bring about a recession of the disorder, or at least to keep it under control. The most common example we have of this procedure is the uterine fibroid tumour.

All the disorders and all the problems to which I have referred will be fully dealt with in their respective chapters. Appropriately the next four chapters will be concerned with young girls and their problems.

## 2

## YOUR SMALL DAUGHTER

If nature has her way our young daughters of today will become the mothers of tomorrow. This is why nature has brought it about that all of us of the animal kingdom, whether we be humans or of lower degree, and normal, have a powerful instinct to love and cherish our daughters from the time they are born and onwards. Of course the same applies to our sons, who may one day become fathers, but biologically the girls are more important than the boys for they possess, or will possess, not only the cells which when brought together will initiate new life, as do the boys, but, in addition, they possess those most intricate and delicate organs which make it possible one day to nourish and bring to maturity this new life.

To witness the loving care and devotion of mothers (and fathers) lavished upon their children can be a deeply moving experience. Living as we do in a world torn with strife and dissension, seething with hate and eaten up with materialism it is comforting to be made aware that to love is a basic instinct inherent in all of us.

Since the welfare of women is the be-all and end-all of my calling I am, of course, more closely involved in caring for girls, but much of the counsel I shall give will be applicable to the young of both sexes. The care of our children must begin at the time of conception for it is within the mother's womb that the foundations of good health and vigour are laid down. When the women we are treating become pregnant we practitioners are presented with a wonderful opportunity of ensuring that everything is done to preserve and fortify the health of the mother-to-be and the baby within her.

The regime at this stage should be so organized that the expectant mother will visit her practitioner at regular intervals for treatment and discussion, especially if it is a first pregnancy. Frequency of visits will depend on the circumstances of the patient and the availability of the practitioner but the intervals should not be greater than four weeks. Between times the practitioner can, of course, be contacted by letter or telephone when advice about some problem is desired.

My own procedure, in addition to directing what the dietary regime should be, is to give my charge a special form of osteopathic treatment followed by simple breathing and pelvic exercises. This promotes the circulation and improves the functioning of the parts of the body and, in particular, the reproductive organs.

## Restrictions During Pregnancy

The dietary regime should be designed to ensure that the mother-to-be is adequately nourished but at the same time, does not put on weight in the usual places. The total permissible gain in weight during the course of pregnancy, taking into account the baby itself, the fluid-filled capsule in which it develops and the placenta, and also the growth of the breasts, should not greatly exceed twenty pounds. The foetal child is very susceptible to the dietary indiscretions of the mother and can be adversely influenced thereby, as we appreciate when we consider an extreme example such as that of the thalidomide tragedy when a large number of grossly deformed babies were born because the mothers had taken the drug. During pregnancy strong spices, condiments, and alcohol should be strictly limited, whilst drugs should be avoided altogether. Smoking should be given up. If medicines are required they should be restricted to herbal or homoeopathic remedies. It should be mentioned in passing that these restrictions are applicable also during the time a baby is breast-fed. X-rays can endanger the welfare of the baby, especially during the first three or four months of pregnancy.

In the course of taking care of a large number of women during their pregnancy I have been particularly impressed with the benefit that has been derived from taking a balanced course of natural vitamins, together with essential minerals, especially calcium. All the mothers have done well and the babies have been healthy, vigorous and good-tempered.

When the age of ten is reached serious consideration should be given to taking your daughter to a practitioner for a physical check-up. If you are fortunate in having the right kind of G.P. who understands children and is conscious of the vulnerability of girls, in particular, and is not pressed for time, he could serve your purpose very well but if, as is the case with many of my readers, you are accustomed to being looked after by a medical herbalist and/or naturopath, then he too must fulfil the same conditions, otherwise you are not likely to get much satisfaction in your solicitude for your daughter.

Some mothers will think that the periodical examination of children carried out by the school medical officer is sufficient but, unfortunately, this is usually so cursory that only gross anatomical defects are likely to be detected.

At this point I must go back somewhat in order to tell you how it can be brought about that this physical examination will be a pleasurable and exciting event for your daughter and not a dreadful ordeal which she will not wish to repeat.

From the earliest age both boys and girls should be brought up to be proud of their bodies and not ashamed of them. This kind of shame is a relic of the Victorian era when there were such extremes of prudery as seeing that little girls were carefully cloaked up to the moment of stepping into a bath and immediately on getting out of it. There can be no doubt that, within reason, nudity is entirely natural and wholesome in children from babyhood upwards. Your daughter will be far more likely to grow up to be health-conscious and healthy if she is an outright exhibitionist, than if she has been so inhibited that to expose her body is a dreadful ordeal.

The result of upbringing will at once be clear when your daughter is taken to a practitioner for her first complete physical check-up. The examination will be difficult to carry out, and of limited value, if your daughter is embarrassed and uncoöperative but of maximum benefit if she looks upon it as an exciting adventure and is proud of her body and its development, and hopeful that she will win praise when she is under examination.

In the course of the examination the height/weight ratio, with allowance for body build, will give a good indication of the nutritional status of your daughter and provide an opportunity to discuss her diet. Owing to the partiality of children to carbohydrates she is likely to be over-weight rather than under-weight.

The training of children in their eating habits is a delicate matter. Whether your efforts be frustrating or rewarding is to some extent unpredictable but much depends on the nature of your relationship with your children.

**Different Ideas About Diet**

Although in agreement in most things,  it sometimes happens

that parents have different ideas about diet. In these cases one usually finds that the mother is the more diet-conscious, tending to lean towards food reform and vegetarianism whilst the father scornfully rejects what he looks upon as cranky ideas and goes along gaily with the conventional dietary habits he and his fellow men have always been accustomed to. This situation presents a real problem and one in which the couple ought to make a great effort to reconcile their differences. Given the bond of affection we would expect to prevail, and the overriding concern of both parents for their common welfare as a family, it ought to be possible for the nutritionally conscious one to convert the other. After all, there is an abundance of literature available in support of a truly wholesome and nutritious diet. To stray briefly from the point; one of the saddest of present-day happenings is that in which sudden death overtakes men of middle age. Often they fall dead in the street, in their mid-forties, when they believed themselves to be in perfect health. These disasters are usually due to coronary thrombosis, a disease acknowledged to result mainly from over-indulgence in a rich and unwholesome diet. Any woman who can convert her husband to become a food reformist for the sake of their children may, at the same time, have taken the momentous step, quite incidentally, that will go far to ensure that she will not become an early widow. Ideally, couples should settle once and for all any differences they may have about their way of life before their children arrive.

Where diet and nutrition are concerned one of the most difficult problems parents may have to face is to prevent their children from developing a craze for carbohydrates. Outside influences are overwhelming. When the musical chimes of the ice-cream van are heard in the neighbourhood children in many households automatically expect to be given money in response to the invitation 'stop me and buy one'. How some parents must curse this imposition! Usually it is the done thing for visitors to bring sweets for the children. At the earliest age many children, as a result of the unwise indulgence of their parents, will develop a sweet tooth. The school tuck shop will be more conspicuous for sweets than anything else. It is not surprising that it has become common for two-year-olds to be fitted with false teeth, as we were told at an annual conference of the British Dental Association. Mothers were blamed for giving children too many sweets and sugary snacks. The problem does not offer an easy solution but from an early age children should be given apples and other fruit in preference to sweets and parents should set an example by denying themselves confectionery and severely restricting their intake of sugar. Their own health will also benefit. To a lesser degree, over-consumption of salt is common in families. The custom of automatically sprinkling salt on every savoury dish will certainly be copied by children if their parents follow it and it will be to their detriment. A craving for both sugar and salt is easily acquired but, fortunately, with the exercise of self-discipline the craving is fairly easy to overcome. Lose no time in setting about it if you have children. Whilst we are on this subject I should like to add that another unhealthy indulgence parents would do well to abandon, if they have children, is smoking.

When we left the subject of physical examination we did so to discuss the relationship of the dietary regime to the height/weight ratio. After remarking that if you permit your children to become overweight for their age it will be an indication that they are having an excess of carbohydrates in their diet, we will return to the examination.

The condition of the hair as well as that of the teeth will be a reflection of the quality of a child's diet. If it is dry, brittle and lustreless there is likely to be a deficiency of vitamins, especially A and B-complex and perhaps also of calcium  A reliable multi-vitamin/mineral tablet coupled with the inclusion of more food containing these elements will be the best answer.

## Posture

It is regrettably common in girls to have round shoulders and a poking head, and again I must blame parents for letting their children become over-prudish. When girls become conscious that their breasts are growing they should be filled with pride and satisfaction that this is so and not be ashamed to let the world take note of their development. Once the stooping habit is acquired, in an attempt to hide the breasts, it can take years of remedial exercises to regain a good posture.

A small degree of lateral curvature of the spine can be accepted but if it is sufficient to be obvious to the untrained eye something will have to be done about it. It will almost certainly be due to one leg being shorter than the other. The hip on the low side will be lower and the shoulder on the same side will be higher. This condition will present an orthopaedic problem involving the provision of a built-up shoe on the low side.

Hollow back (lordosis) often accompanies round shoulders. Pelvic inclination will be excessive and the tone of the abdominal and buttock muscles will be poor. Both conditions can be corrected by teaching suitable exercises. If these are carried out conscientiously and correctly a gratifying improvement in posture will be the reward.

Narrow hips in a girl must be looked upon as a disadvantage. It will present a problem in later years when she is called upon to bear children. Fortunately there are again exercises which improve the condition not, of course, by making the pelvis larger, as this would be an impossibility, but by making it more flexible.

We do not see knock-knees and bow-legs often in these days, when there is little gross malnutrition, but these defects should be looked for. If they exist suitable exercises must be prescribed and taught.

Foot trouble is more common, but again less so than it used to be, now that sensible shoes for children are readily available. Children should be encouraged to walk about in bare feet in the house and on the lawn in summer time. This enables the feet to develop in the way nature intended and thus there will be less likelihood of fallen arches later on. You will be confronted with a problem when your daughter reaches an age when she wants something more elegant than school shoes, with high heels and pointed toes. This is when the trouble starts, so you must try hard to let the transition be gradual and not too drastic. Point out that pointed toes spell bunions, whilst high heels may do the same and, in addition, give rise to aches and pains if she walks far. Incidentally, please do encourage your girls to walk whenever they can. An untold amount of harm occurs to women gynaecologically because they walk far too little from childhood upwards, preferring to ride about in motor cars and other vehicles.

In the gynaecological sphere there is usually little to look for in a pre-adolescent girl. A casual examination of the vulva coupled with information you as her mother can provide, will show if there is any soreness or any discharge. The only disorders likely to occur are vulvovaginitis and bartholinitis, both of which can be contracted through carelessness when using public lavatories.

Girls should be trained to always put toilet paper on the seat of a public lavatory before using it.

If you, yourself, become aware that your daughter has a discharge because she has told you so, or because you have noticed it on her underwear, you should lose no time in taking her to see a practitioner, preferably one likely to prescribe herbal or homoeopathic remedies. Doctors are far too ready to prescribe antibiotics for children, in spite of being frequently warned by their own profession that they should not do so.

Malposition of the uterus, which is all too common in mature women, and often the cause of considerable suffering, to say nothing of infertility, can usually be traced to childhood indiscretions. The most common is the tendency for young girls to go far too long without emptying their bladders, either because of shyness or through lack of opportunity. The resulting pressure on the developing uterus is almost certain to bring about an early retroversion.

Constipation is another bugbear causing unnatural pressure in the opposite direction, which spells antiflexion. It is imperative that you train your daughter in such a way that she will not develop constipation because if she does, not only may it endanger the well-being of her uterus but her entire health, both general and gynaecological, for the rest of her days will be in jeopardy.

It is often said that strenuous exercise is the cause of malposition of the uterus in young girls but with this theory I cannot agree. I am of the opinion that a reasonable amount of exercise, as in running, jumping and playing tennis, hockey and netball, is far more likely to promote a well-positioned uterus than the reverse. This is because the ligaments which support the organ are more likely to maintain their proper tone through being exercised than would be the case if your girl leads an over-sedentary life.

It is not possible in one chapter to advise you how to take care of your daughters beyond the pre-adolescent stage. This being the case, I propose to give you my views about the upbringing of adolescents and teenagers in the next chapter.

## 3

# THE TEENAGE GIRL

Those of us who haye adolescent daughters or are concerned with the welfare of young girls are perplexed by the rapid growth in recent years of what has come to be called 'permissiveness', meaning, in other words, sexual freedom.

In this permissive society many of our leaders, including not a few politicians, regard permissiveness as progress towards a higher form of civilization. This, presumably, means that there is merit in giving people more freedom to select their own standards of self-expression and behaviour and to adhere to these without censure from neighbours or sanctions imposed by existing authorities. Inevitably there comes a point, however, at which society must take stock of the effects of change and decide whether the results of permissiveness are doing damage to individuals and society as a whole.

Of all the aspects of human behaviour none requires more careful consideration than the relations between the sexes, leading — as they are liable to do — to the production of new life and to profound emotional relationships on which depend the stability of families and thus of the whole social structure. Such a consideration will lead to an assessment of the implications of divorce, of broken homes, of illegitimacy, of abortions, of delinquency, of various psychiatric problems and of other matters which permissiveness has brought in its train, including the very alarming one of the worldwide recrudescence of venereal disease among the young.

Despite modern methods of control, we are informed in a leading article in *The Lancet* of 1st August 1970 that this new outbreak of venereal disease is causing anxiety.

## Increase in Gonorrhoea
In an article in *The Sunday Times* of 9th August in the same year we learn that in the United Kingdom the figures for gonorrhoea (the most common venereal disease) alone show an annual increase of 17 per cent. It is sad to relate that the biggest single group in which the infection occurs includes girls between fifteen and nineteen years of age. The suggested

explanation for this is that anti-social urges among young girls manifest mainly as promiscuity. The ever-willing teenage girl is the female equivalent of the skinhead in bovver boots. Although the menace of V.D. is bad enough in this country, it is far worse in countries where permissiveness is even more advanced than with us. Sweden has four times as much gonorrhoea per head of population as Britain, whilst the United States had 1½ million cases last year, a third of them teenagers. The American Social Health Association reported to their government this year that gonorrhoea was 'by the most conservative estimate clearly out of control'.

Dr Bill Jones, Secretary-General of the Health Education Council (Britain) was quoted in *The Daily Telegraph* of 2nd June 1970 as follows:

> V.D. is increasing rapidly, and more rapidly in girls than boys. This must mean that girls are more promiscuous than boys.
>
> The increase in women is very disturbing because the disease takes much longer to show in women. Whereas a man will have obvious symptoms within ten days a woman can be in complete ignorance for months. In fact they often come for treatment after their boy friends have consulted us.

*The Lancet* article, already quoted, says that those, including members of the medical profession, who make light of the increasing tendency of young people to experiment with sex before marriage, and even encourage them to do so, must consider the implications carefully. Complications of V.D. are common and include pelvic infections in women, sometimes resulting in severe illness, prolonged anxiety and unhappiness, and sterility.

I have written at length on the subject of venereal disease as a preliminary to a discussion of sex education because V.D. has now become a matter that should on no account be evaded, even though it is unpleasant.

From the earliest age questions asked by children, whether they concern sex or any other subject, should be answered truthfully and as fully as the age capacity of the child warrants. There should be no more inhibition in answering questions about matters appertaining to sex than about history, geography, astronomy or cooking. If this has become the custom it will make the task of the practitioner much easier if at any time he is called upon to treat your daughter for some gynaecological disorder or to carry out a physical examination at the age of ten or so, as I advocated in the previous chapter on this subject.

Whether or not this physical check-up at the age of ten-plus has been carried out, it certainly ought to be laid on at the age of, say, fourteen, especially if physical development appears to be retarded or if there has been no indication that menstruation will soon occur or if menstruation has already taken place and has been painful or unsatisfactory in other respects.

If it is (unhappily) the case that you have not been able to freely discuss 'the facts of life' with your daughter and you have reason to think she has acquired the knowledge in an unsatisfactory manner at school or from other girls the opportunity should be taken to make good the omission at the time of the examination.

The question will arise whether you should be present or not. In the case of teenage girls I always ask the question 'would you like to come with your mother or by yourself?' The proportion of those who wish to come alone and those with mother is about equal but in the case of girls who are known to be ill-informed about the essentials of sex education this part of the session ought to be private. If you, as the girl's mother, have been unable to talk freely to your daughter before taking her to a practitioner for a check-up it would clearly cause much embarrassment if you were present at a time when he was trying to gain your daughter's confidence and produce an atmosphere favourable for a serious talk.

When it comes to a physical examination the legal aspect of the matter must be considered. It used to be the custom for a nurse to be present in the room whenever a female of any age was examined by a male practitioner, no matter whether he was orthodox or unorthodox. This custom has, by common consent, been modified or abandoned in recent years, partly because it is recognized as a relic of a more prudish and suspicious era and partly on grounds of expense. In the house in which my consulting room was situated when this was written there are usually as many as five practitioners of various categories working in different rooms. If each had a nurse in attendance the overhead costs, already very great, and ever on the increase, would be much higher. To keep our fees at a reasonable level we have to economize where we can. It is sufficient to have one receptionist always within easy reach of any part of the building. Girls of sixteen or over can and often do, without causing any legal complications, arrange their own appointments and request a consultation which would involve a physical examination without a third party being actually present in the same room. In the present article I am considering girls of an earlier age and would advise that during that part of the consultation in which a physical examination is necessary the girl's mother should be present but the session should not end without the girl being given an opportunity to have a private talk with the practitioner.

## Abortion Horror

The matter of venereal disease has been fully covered. Another matter which should be included in the practitioner's talk is that of contraception. On quite a few occasions when young girls have been brought to me by their mothers for examination and I have found them to be pregnant, I have been amazed at the total disregard there has been of contraception. Whether we like it or not we have to face the fact that the times have changed dramatically and that promiscuity among teenagers has become alarmingly common. Even though recent legislation has made it fairly easy for pregnancy in a young girl to be terminated, the whole business fills many of us, including doctors and nurses, with horror. Because they are women there is something particularly harrowing to sensitive nurses in abortion operations, especially when carried out in advanced stages of pregnancy. The dedicated among them were called to their profession by a desire to help in reducing the sufferings of humanity and the saving of lives. In abortions they see the anthithesis of the latter ideal. As for the former, they are aware that in some hospitals deserving gynaecological cases are being put back in a waiting list already two years long or more, to make room for abortions. These include women who cannot have babies and others who are in pain. It was reported not long ago that at a hospital in Lancashire all abortions were halted due to a boycott by the operating theatre staff. Doctors in the area were obliged to put abortion patients on waiting lists elsewhere.

Once again I must use that well-worn dictum, prevention is better than cure. We should not try to hide from ourselves the fact that the sexual urge is immensely strong, especially in the young, and do nothing. If we, who constitute society, have been unable to curb the stimulation of this instinct in the young whom we see all around us we should, at least, do something towards providing antidotes when we are in a position to do so.

Obviously, the best form of prevention lies in the bringing up of our daughters; in setting them a good example and instilling in them a proper appreciation of the fundamentals of a stable society and, in particular, the sanctity of marriage and the undesirability of anticipating the rewards that marriage ought to bring. They should be encouraged to belong to organizations with wholesome principles, such as the Girl Guides. All that need be said about religious teaching is that the decline in this has undoubtedly contributed to the sad decline in moral integrity we are now witnessing. Children should be encouraged to attend Sunday Schools and to take religion seriously.

### The Pill: 'Potential Time-Bomb'

When girls go to colleges and universities they are likely to find that permissiveness is the order of the day and recognized by the authorities. Here the prevention of pregnancy has become a matter of economics. University education is a costly business and to have a girl's course of study interrupted or brought to an end by a mishap of this kind must be avoided if possible. Thus, advice about contraception by the resident doctor is freely available. Unfortunately, the method of choice is 'the pill'. As readers will become aware, I have consistently condemned the use of the pill because of its potential damage to gynaecological integrity and general health. Since it is fully covered in Chapter Twenty-One I need say no more here about the pill beyond quoting an American cancer research specialist, who has told a United States Senate Committee that the pill is 'a potential time-bomb with a twenty-year fuse'. When the circumstances appear to warrant it I tell girls with whose welfare I am concerned that in the event of the sexual urge becoming too strong to resist they must make absolutely certain that their partner uses a sheath. This is not usually regarded as the ideal form of contraception for married couples but it has the advantage of not only being almost 100 per cent safe if properly used, but it is also a reliable safeguard against contracting venereal disease.

In the previous chapter on the same subject, when the welfare of younger girls was discussed, I explained that whether a physical examination is going to be a painful ordeal or a pleasurable and exciting event is likely to depend a great deal on upbringing. From the earliest age boys and girls should be encouraged to be proud of their bodies and not ashamed of them. There can be no doubt that, within reason, nudity is entirely natural and wholesome in children from babyhood upwards. Let me repeat, your daughter will be far more likely to grow up to be health-conscious and healthy if she is an outright exhibitionist than if she has been so inhibited that to expose her body is a dreadful ordeal.

We are now concerned with adolescent girls, and their physical examination will present no problem if it has been the custom to take them to your practitioner annually for a check-up from the age of ten or thereabouts. In those who come for the first time when they are teenagers the effect of upbringing will be at once apparent. The examination will be difficult to carry out and of limited value if your daughter is embarrassed and uncoöperative but of maximum benefit if she looks upon it as an exciting adventure and is proud of her body and its development, and is hopeful she will win praise when she is under observation.

There is no need to repeat what I have said in the previous chapter about a general examination as there should now be more emphasis on the gynaecological aspect of the matter.

In the last two decades it has been found that, on the whole, girls begin to menstruate at an earlier age than used to be the case. Fourteen was once the average age of menstruation to commence but twelve is now quite common. In early developers menstruation can begin as early as ten whilst in late developers there need be no cause for concern if nothing has happened by the age of fourteen.

I shall deal at length in other chapters with the treatment of lack of menstruation and menstrual disorders in young girls and will not, therefore, say anything further here but if there has been no menstruation at fifteen or if it has started previously and then stopped or if it is painful, you should most certainly make an appointment for your daughter to be attended to by a practitioner likely to be conversant with these problems.

### Vaginal Examination

During the routine examination of a young girl, as, for example, when there is pain in the lower part of the abdomen, a bimanual rectoabdominal examination is nearly always sufficient and satisfactory. However, there must be no hesitation about making a vaginal examination when it is indicated in cases of vaginal soreness or discharge, abnormal bleeding, pelvic pain and other suspicious symptoms. Many girls now use vaginal tampons of some kind at an early age and in these it is quite easy to insert a well-lubricated index finger without causing pain. With experience, as much information can be obtained by means of a one-finger examination as when two fingers are used. In girls with a very small and sensitive hymenal opening it may be possible to dilate it gently so that it will admit a single finger if one first uses a local anaesthetic followed by adequate lubrication. Before an examination is made of any virgin the practitioner should explain to the patient, and also to her mother, that there is no need for objection to making a pelvic examination because the lack of an intact hymen is by no means a sign that there has been intercourse, in these days when so many girls experiment with tampons even if they do not use them regularly.

After the vaginal examination has been made, the lower extremities should be observed for varicose veins, swollen ankles, excessive hair growth and deformities. After this the patient is asked to stand so that her back and posture may be examined. In cases where the breasts show signs of becoming unduly large and lacking in tone, advice should be given about the kind of brassière that should be worn, also, suitable exercises should be recommended.

I have found that young girls tend to be unduly worried if they have a vaginal discharge and for this reason something should be said to put the matter in the right perspective. A slight discharge of the consistency of raw white of egg and colourless is quite normal but it may be sufficient to show on the underclothing and may be pale yellow in colour when it dries.

At times the discharge may become thicker and more copious but it may then indicate nothing more serious than a catarrhal condition which is liable to overtake any of the openings of the body lined with mucous membrane when there is a chill or a temporary infection. In this case the discharge can be likened to a catarrhal cold.

In the event of the increased discharge not diminishing after a few days and becoming yellow or green in colour and causing soreness and itching at the entrance of the vagina and adjourning area, there is likely to be some kind of infection.

The two most likely causes which bring about an abnormal discharge and cause local soreness and severe itching in the area, are bacterial infections. They have the Latin names *trichomonas vaginalis* and *candida albicans*. The latter is commonly known as a vaginal 'thrush'. More serious discharges, having some blood or muco-pus mixed up with them and causing external tenderness and discomfort but no itching, could be due to inflammation of the vagina or 'erosion' of the cervix or to gonorrhoea.

Abnormal discharges and itching frequently arise in women and girls of all ages and we do not know precisely how they come about. Fortunately, they can be cured by the use of a therapeutic jelly injected internally, and treatment with homoeopathic remedies. The latter are important and if ignored the infection is liable to recur soon after the injections, after giving temporary relief, are given up. The treatment of vaginal infections is dealt with in greater detail in Chapter Five.

Although taking care of your daughters has occupied two chapters of this book, the subject is clearly so important and complex that to cover it adequately would need the space of an entire volume.

I have endeavoured to cover the most serious problems confronting young girls and those that are most common. I advise parents to let their daughters read the chapters, the first one is for younger girls and both are for teenage girls.

## 4

## THE YOUNG GIRL'S PROBLEMS

A letter I chanced to read in *The Lancet*, and a television feature, drew my attention to a comparatively new development in publishing: the magazine for the teenage girl. In *The Lancet* letter, a doctor expressed the opinion that at least one of these magazines performed a valuable social service by publishing letters received in confidence from teenage girls about some personal problem, together with the solution thought to be appropriate.

I was already aware of the need for a service of this kind because, from time to time among my considerable mail received from readers of *Here's Health*, there are similar letters, not necessarily concerned with a purely gynaecological problem.

Before commenting on the content of these letters to magazines it is desirable to point out that the writers, for the most part, are in a distinct category since this is made clear in the letters themselves. The writers are often extremely worried by their problem and, in some cases, desperately so, but are so placed that they cannot bring themselves to discuss it with one or other of their parents or with the family doctor. Expressions constantly used are 'I am much too embarrassed to ask my mother'; 'You are the only one I can turn to, as my parents would kill me if they knew'; 'I would be so embarrassed and ashamed of this, I would never go to the doctor'; 'I cannot go to my family doctor as he is a close friend of the family'; 'Please do not tell me to visit my doctor because I just couldn't'; 'Please do not answer this letter because I do not want my parents to know, so could you please print this soon because I am desperate'; 'I cannot go to the doctor because he is my father.'

As one would expect, young boys seldom write to these magazines, although a good many are likely to read them with not a little salacious interest, considering that a lot of the letters are very frank, leaving little to the imagination.

One boy was worried because he had a lisp and was advised to go to his family doctor and ask for a letter to the nearest hospital which has a speech therapy unit.

Another boy, aged fifteen, was worried because he was not attracted by girls, preferring the company of other boys. He seemed to fear he might be homosexual. In a sensible reply it was pointed out that adolescence — the period of growing up from childhood to adulthood — is a very confusing time during which people learn how to live as an adult. It is not at all unusual for boys to feel as he did but in the majority of cases it is only a passing phase. He was given the telephone number of the Samaritans and advised to get in touch with that organiz ation if the problem persisted.

An interesting point about this letter was that he was encouraged to write to the magazine because the girls in his class at school often read it and talked about its helpfulness in offering solutions for their problems.

The significance of this is that for every girl who writes to the magazine to seek a solution for her problem there must be dozens with similar problems who find a solution by simply reading the magazine.

## Revolutionary Changes

Those of us likely to be called upon to assist the young in overcoming their difficulties have a duty to keep abreast of the times and adjust our thinking and our attitude from time to time. We have to recognize that revolutionary changes have taken place since the Victorian or Edwardian eras in which we were born. Because, in the letters they write, teenagers are able to express their feelings and explain their problems far more freely than they could in speech, face to face with another person, these letters have a unique value in giving us a reliable insight into what the female teenagers' personal problems are and how they are behaving in their relationship with the opposite sex.

In my capacity as gynaecologist, it is my custom always to take an interest in the children of my patients, and the girls in particular, since they are more directly within my sphere.

As a matter of course, girls with menstrual or other gynaecological disorders come to see me either on their own accord or are brought by their mothers, but it happens not infrequently that other problems arise. There can be much misunderstanding and friction and even rebellion.

Only last week, with the exercise of great tact, a mother was able to persuade her daughter, aged fourteen, to come along to have a talk. The case was somewhat similar to one which gave rise to a letter to one of the magazines starting: 'I am 15 and I used to love my father, but now I hate him.' In the reply it was pointed out that the transition from utterly dependent, adoring childhood to capable, independent, but still friendly and affectionate, adulthood, can be a very difficult one giving rise to conflicting emotions.

When the impulse to be cheeky and rebellious cannot be controlled, an early opportunity should be taken after an outburst to apologise to father, telling him you don't know what comes over you, and growing up is difficult. Most fathers will respond with sympathy and understanding. I agree with this reply.

The letters reveal a surprising lack of biological knowledge among teenage girls, thus questions are quite frequently asked about breast development, hair distribution and the external genital area.

Ailments concerning which advice is sought include menstrual failure, menstrual irregularity, vaginal discharge and irritation, venereal disease and overweight. In reply the writers are, invariably, advised, quite rightly to consult their family doctor but, as I have already pointed out, many for various reasons, do not like doing this. All I can say is that it is sad that this should be the case.

### Relations with Boyfriends

A great many of the letters concern relations with boyfriends, and from these it is clear that promiscuity is widespread among girls from the age of fourteen upwards. Some of the writers make no bones about their sexual relations and seek advice on contraception. Others are afraid they might have contracted venereal disease and wonder what they should do. In all cases, the advice given is down-to-earth and practical and no attempt is made to moralize except in blatant cases of loose behaviour.

Perhaps the most interesting letters, in that they show the other side of the picture from all-too-ready promiscuity, are those from girls who are hesitant. One of these reads roughly as follows: 'My boyfriend has recently asked me to make love to him but, as we are only 15, I feel it would be wrong. I like my boyfriend very much and don't want to lose him but I am afraid if I don't give in he will chuck me. I have talked it over with him and he says I am being stupid. Is there some means of meeting him halfway?'

To such letters the reply is unvaried and emphatic. A boy who uses this kind of blackmail is not interested in a good relationship but only in sex. If what the girl wants is real love she will not get it by 'buying' it with a sexual compliance she doesn't really feel.

Sometimes the answer is differently worded but the meaning is the same. If a boy will only stay with a girl if she lets him have intercourse with her, he isn't worth having. Sooner or later he will drop her anyway, since he will have no respect for her. This is a good way of putting it because mutual respect is the strongest link a couple can have.

We may think that in an age in which sex matters are so freely discussed and written about, there would be no thirst for knowledge. That this is not the case is revealed by the letters we are discussing. This one is rather pathetic. 'I am 15 and have no one to turn to; my mother is 50 and I just cannot talk to her about my problem as we do not get on well together and I am an only child. Some of the things the girls say at school are frightening. Because of this I am afraid to go out with boys. Please can you help me?'

She was advised to approach a favourite schoolteacher or write for a list of suitable books to read on sex education and boy/girl relationships. The reply would have to be sent to an address other than that of her home.

## Sex Education and Delinquency

The ideas of doctors, psychologists and sociologists vary enormously about what should constitute sex education. At one extreme we have Dr Louise Eickhoff, a child psychologist of Birmingham, who contends that sex education is responsible for the rise in sex delinquency. In her survey 40 per cent of girls were delinquent after receiving sex instruction and she claims that such education had lowered the peak age for delinquency in girls from 16 to 15. In her report to the Secretary of State for Education, she states that the kind of sex education many teenagers receive destroys adolescence and plunges the child into adult sex knowledge, adult urges and cravings before the child's system of self-discipline is correspondingly strong.

At the other extreme we have *The Little Red Schoolbook*, the publishers of which were found guilty in a magistrates' court under the law relating to obscene literature. This meant that publication of the book was banned and rightly so. In a liberal use of four-letter words teenagers were encouraged to indulge in sexual intercourse if they felt like it. In the book a great deal was also written about the rights of pupils and how to secure them by organizing demonstrations and walkouts. Very mischievous.

At this extreme we have also had Dr Martin Cole's sex film called *Growing Up*, which gave rise to a storm of protest when an attempt was made to have it shown in schools. There was much in the film to which even the most liberal took exception, in particular the appearance of a young schoolteacher naked and in the act of masturbating.

The film was not actually banned but, like *The Little Red Schoolbook*, having had its fling in the newspapers, the public for the most part will have forgotten it by now.

Very much with us is the Reverend Chad Varah, Rector of St Stephen's, Walbrook, in the City of London, married with five children and two grandchildren and founder and Director of the Samaritans. He is, at present, in the process of launching a new movement to be called Christian Lib., which will preach the gospel of rationality. He writes, 'We already have more than three-quarters of the population turned against God and His Church because the official teaching of the Church about sex makes God less loving and understanding than many humans.' Also, 'We have no right to say "by the age of 14 you should/should not have done so-and-so." It depends on the individual teenager and on his or her circumstances. What we can, and must, say is that approaches to the opposite sex are to be encouraged and not condemned. What is important is not what has been done at what age, but whether the teenager is a loving and understanding person, literally feeling his or her way towards good personal relationships.'

There seems to be little doubt that the Samaritans do good work in helping teenagers who are in difficulties and at least one of the magazines with which I opened this discussion recommends contacting the organizations in appropriate cases.

At least twenty books about sex education have been written in recent years and among them it is not easy to find one that steers the middle course, which I think is what we need.

One of the latest publications enjoys the authority of the British Medical Association and was written by a woman doctor. Having regard for today's more liberal outlook, I think it can claim to be moderate.

Unfortunately, many parents who might have felt inclined to give the booklet to their teenage children to read instead of themselves expounding on the facts of life, would be put off so doing by the crudeness of the identical front and back covers. No useful purpose is served by printing the single word 'Sex' in huge letters right in the middle of the covers.

### Sex Requires Education

If children could be adequately taught by merely giving them books to read there would be no need for lessons once the ability to read had been acquired. Like any other subject, sex for its proper understanding requires elucidation and discussion as well as the provision of text books and this seems to bring us to the crux of the whole situation. Who should do the teaching?

Although there are outstanding exceptions, schoolteachers for the most part are ill-equipped to do the job, having none of the necessary qualifications, and with teachers there is no certainty that they will keep to the middle of the road.

Among doctors, the average National Health general practitioner is hard put to give his patients more than five minutes of his time in an interview and cannot be seriously considered for a task requiring hours rather than minutes to perform successfully. The private practitioner or the unorthodox practitioner, if suitably equipped, might be a better proposition.

The clergy have more time than doctors and from that point of view could do good work, but the Reverend Chad Varah's Christian Lib. Movement has a very long way to go before more than a few persons are likely to have acquired what is now thought to be the right attitude.

Our best hope, without doubt, remains with parents and, as time goes on, the situation should steadily improve. The teenagers of today who have, through the right kind of teaching acquired a liberal outlook towards sex and its implications, will be well equipped to impart the same knowledge in a straightforward and uninhibited manner to their sons and daughters when they are married. They will do so with enthusiasm because they, themselves, will have derived immense benefit from having had their marriage enriched as a result of their knowledge.

We hear much about the lack of communication and

understanding between the parents of today and their teenage children and I am in no doubt that this is largely due to circumstances arising from their differing attitude to sex. Most parents will have been brought up in an age when sex was not a subject that could be openly discussed. Often their parents were too inhibited to impart even the elements of sexual knowledge to them. Thus they, themselves, gaining their knowledge from school mates in the same situation, the blind leading the blind as it were, acquired the same furtive attitude. This situation is clearly disclosed in many of the letters written by teenage girls to the magazines under discussion.

It is never too late to mend. Parents, or would-be parents, who have had this kind of upbringing, have a duty to set about discarding their inhibitions and, at the same time, educating themselves through reading a few of the many books on sex education now available. As I have pointed out, these differ considerably and some are extreme. The middle course is the one that should provide the foundation of parents' relationship with their children.

The duty of teaching teenage girls should not be confined to mothers. It is of great importance in the development of girls, and their future ability to make a good adjustment in marriage, that they should have a loving, confident and uninhibited relationship with their fathers and be able to discuss their private problems just as freely with him as with their mother.

Most important of all is the need to make it abundantly clear to teenagers of both sexes that, having acquired an education in sex, it is up to them to use their knowledge in a sensible manner and not make the fatal mistake of getting involved in sordid and loveless experimentation.

It cannot be too strongly impressed upon the teenagers to whom it is our privilege to impart sexual knowledge that with knowledge there must be responsibility. More important than the teaching of sex is the teaching of the significance of love, love in the fullest meaning of the word, love which includes respect, responsibility, foresight, patience, kindness, restraint, constancy and faithfulness.

The debasement of the sexual relationship — teenage sex for 'kicks' without love, having sex because it is the done thing — is all too liable to stunt the emotions to such a degree that the truly loving relationship which is, perhaps, the most precious and rewarding thing attainable by a man and a woman will not be forthcoming. They have thrown away the substance for the shadow.

Promiscuity has another aspect. Professor Sir John Stallworthy, one of our most experienced and distinguished gynaecologists, in his paper presented at the Health Congress at Eastbourne in April 1972, had this to say concerning teenage promiscuous experience:

> Recent studies show there is a disquietingly high incidence of changes in the epithelium [cellular substance of the mucous membrane; in this case the vagina is presumed], recognised in older age groups to be associated with a higher risk of the development of cancer. The young who are not aware of these dangers cannot be considered as irresponsible, simply because their actions expose them to these increased risks. But surely those of us who are aware of the hazards are irresponsible if we fail to issue the necessary warnings.

Among the magazines catering for teenage girls are *Petticoat*, *19* and *Honey*. Anne Edwards, writing for *The Sunday Telegraph*, criticizes all three for taking part in what is described as 'the boldest consumer advertising campaign yet' for contraceptives. Most of the letters quoted appeared in *Petticoat*.

The question-and-answer page in *Woman* is also deservedly popular with teenagers.

## 5

## CHILDHOOD GYNAECOLOGICAL PROBLEMS

Although rare it sometimes happens that the sexual organs of a newborn baby deviate in some way or other from normal. When such defects exist in the external genital structures they will be apparent when the baby is inspected. It may be that the clitoris, which in a girl is the counterpart of the penis in the male, is large enough to actually resemble a small penis. True hermaphrodites, wherein the characteristics of both sexes are present, are extremely uncommon but it is important when there is some doubt that the true sex of the infant be determined immediately at birth so as to avoid the unhappy consequences of a female being brought up as a male and vice versa.

The thin membrane of tissue partly closing the entrance of the vagina in normal girls and known as the hymen may be unusually thick and have no opening and then we have the imperforate hymen. This will probably cause no difficulty until menstruation begins. Then the flow of blood cannot escape and will cause great distress by accumulating in the vagina. To make sure this will not happen, all female children should be examined gynaecologically a few years before menstruation is likely to occur. The age of ten might be suggested. The defect can easily be rectified by means of a simple operation.

It sometimes happens, though again very rarely, that there is a band of fibrous tissue in the centre of the vagina dividing it into two compartments (septate vagina). Even more rare is the complete absence of a vagina. The septate vagina can be surgically corrected but the creation of an artificial vagina by plastic operation is a much more complicated matter. The uterus may also be abnormal, although this would not be discovered in childhood. Like the septate vagina, it may have two chambers instead of one, with only one cervix. All these conditions of congenital faulty development of the reproductive organs can best be avoided by care on the part of the mother before she becomes pregnant and during pregnancy. There should be sound nutrition properly supervised, and complete avoidance of drugs, including 'the pill' (see Chapters Eight, Nine and Twenty-One) and smoking.

Fortunately, tumours of the reproductive organs are not often found in infancy and childhood. Certain kinds of tumour will stimulate early development of the sexual organs, in which case a girl of eight or younger will undergo the characteristic changes of puberty with the onset of menstruation. Determination of the cause of premature sexual development is clearly important since it may be capable of correction.

The importance of hygiene in the female child from infancy upwards must not be overlooked. Inflammation of the external genital organs is liable to occur if they are not regularly cleansed with warm water and a mild soap, preferably a herbal one. Within the folds of tissue there will be found a white secretion called *smegma* and this will cause irritation if allowed to accumulate excessively. It can easily be removed with a small wad of cotton wool dipped in almond oil. As children grow older, foreign bodies — especially sand in the sea bathing season — may find their way into the vagina and give rise to inflammation with a troublesome vaginal discharge. The assistance of your practitioner should be sought when this is noticed. As soon as they become old enough, little girls should receive proper instruction concerning their personal cleanliness.

## Personality Changes

Changes which culminate in puberty and the capacity for motherhood will begin to occur from the age of ten on average. The girl's body, hitherto similar to that of a boy, will begin to assume more rounded and feminine contours. The breasts will begin to emerge and swell. The vulval folds will become more pronounced and pubic and axillary hair will gradually appear. At this stage personality changes must be anticipated with moodiness, liability to burst into tears with complaints of being misunderstood, and emotional instability in general. Temporarily the girl will inevitably become what we commonly describe as 'difficult'.

These changes are, of course, perfectly natural, since they are the consequences of the action of hormones which are brought into play at this juncture. These take time in establishing a normal pattern of behaviour when full maturity is reached. At the age of ten or thereabouts, or even earlier, one of the parents or some other understanding person who might be more knowledgeable and experienced, should explain the meaning of all these changes before they occur. In most cases the girl's mother is the best person to undertake this talk but sometimes the closeness of the relationship may result in there being an inhibitory barrier which makes the task difficult, with an emotional undertone, when there ought to be a completely frank and matter-of-fact attitude. In such cases it seems a pity that the family practitioner, whether he be orthodox or unorthodox, should not be more regularly called upon to carry out this crucial duty.

The importance of environment in determining a girl's attitude to sexual development is much greater than many of us realize. If menstruation is regarded by her mother as a monthly ordeal — often referred to as 'the curse' — and something that must be endured as an unfair burden on her sex, the effect on her growing daughter can be highly unsatisfactory. The young girl may then regard with dread and resentment the changes in her body she is unable to prevent. How much more wholesome is an attitude which depicts menstruation as something normal and healthy and very much to be desired! Parents have substantial assurance that they have been successful in the upbringing of their daughter, in so far as the sexual sphere is concerned, if she hails the first appearance of menstruation and all the accompanying signs with quiet satisfaction, happy in the thought that she is on the threshold of womanhood.

### Irregular Menstruation

In some girls menstruation will be irregular for the first year or two and may skip several months at a time. The amount and consistency of the flow may also vary a good deal. At first ovulation may not occur at the appointed time each month. This is because the ovarian hormone, progesterone, which exercises control over menstruation, is not present in adequate quantity but the basic reason for this, which is intermittent failure to ovulate, is not necessarily abnormal or uncommon at a time when the cycle is being established in a young girl. However, if there is a succession of heavy periods the loss of blood will almost certainly result in some degree of anaemia. It is appropriate to mention here that naturopaths strongly disapprove of the tendency among medical doctors to prescribe synthetic hormones and iron pills to young girls in these circumstances. The conservative methods for putting matters right, which we naturopaths prefer to employ, will not harm the delicate apparatus provided by nature. This may well happen when drugs are administered, causing permanent damage.

Of course, emotional problems will bring about irregular menstruation in a young girl, as they do in mature women; so also will illness. Going on an exciting holiday will almost certainly delay menstruation.

Dysmenorrhoea, by which is meant painful menstruation, sometimes occurs from the start and when this is so it is liable to continue into adulthood if not successfully treated. If we exclude organic causes such as a misplaced womb or polypoid growths within it and which need specialized treatment, we are left with common, or primary, dysmenorrhoea. The characteristic symptom will be cramp. It will feel as though the womb was refusing to open to expel the products of menstruation, and this will indeed be the case. This type of dysmenorrhoea is a disturbance of function and does not always occur with every menstruation. It may be intermittent. It is most common in highly strung and nervous girls, especially those of excessive sensitivity. The psychological consequences of being conditioned in early childhood to regard menstruation as an illness, or 'being unwell', is much to blame.

The most sensible treatment for this common form of dysmenorrhoea is to give the girl a sympathetic explanation of the entire menstrual process, with emphasis on its naturalness. Your naturopath, if you have one, may be the most competent person to do this and he may at the same time suggest simple exercises for the purpose of bringing about a more healthy condition in the reproductive region in general. If necessary he will prescribe safe and simple herbal or homoeopathic remedies and suggest various methods of alleviating distress when it occurs.

### Douches and Tampons

There is some conflict of opinion about the use of vaginal douches. The custom is common on the continent, less so in this country, but the subject brings to mind the question of sanitary protection and this will be dealt with first. To begin with the ordinary 'towel' will be used but there is a growing tendency for quite young girls to use the tampon type of protection eventually. They are encouraged to do so by advertising and it is known that in boarding schools about half the girls use this form of protection. A lot depends on temperament and sensitivity. The tampon cannot be inserted without preliminary stretching of the hymen and this the girl must do herself, unless a practitioner does it for her. Many are far too sensitive and diffident to go that far and will continue to use the towel. The tampon has advantages when playing games and going for a swim but here I must hasten to add that a swim or a cold bath must not be indulged in earlier than the fourth day of menstruation or serious consequences could result. As a gynaecologist I am not in favour of the regular use of the tampon. It cannot be good for the health of the vagina to keep the waste products of menstruation dammed up for several hours at a time, because the consistency of the natural secretions of the vagina will be adversely influenced thereby. These secretions have an important function in maintaining the vagina and the cervix of the womb in a healthy state. The best advice to give is to use the towel most of the time and reserve the tampon for special occasions. It should never be left in for more than a few hours.

Let us return to the use of vaginal douches. Since the hymenial opening in a virgin is no greater on average than would admit a pencil, some stretching would be necessary before the nozzle of a douche could be inserted. Provided nothing more than water at blood heat is used, and not used too frequently, it could do no harm but the advantage of the custom is not clear. Mothers who wish to encourage their daughters to use the douche should remember that the vagina contains natural secretions, as I have already said, for the protection of its mucous lining and that of the cervix. The composition of this secretion is carefully balanced by nature and slightly acid. Frequent douching would be liable to upset the balance and dilute the secretions and thereby encourage the invasion of parasites such as trichomonas or monilia and that would indeed be a disaster for a young girl. Let us compromise by suggesting that douching with warm water only for hygenic purposes when a period has ceased is permissible. Medicated douches should most certainly not be used excepting under the direction of a practitioner.

This brings me to the end of my fifth chapter. The last four have also been devoted to the problems with which girls are liable to be confronted progressively, from the time they are born until they reach relative maturity. Inevitably there has been a good deal of repetition, especially in regard to the manner in which the mysteries of sex and the implications thereof should be unfolded. We have reached a stage in our evolution at which the very foundations of our society, in which for hundreds of years the keystone has been the marriage that endured, are being shaken by those who tell us that marriage is being outmoded.

All around us we have evidence of how greed and selfishness are slowly but surely bringing about the destruction of the beauties of nature, which have made the world in which we live so wonderful. If — as wise men have told us — civilization contains the seeds of its own destruction, total chaos is what we may be in for. Could anything produce greater chaos than the outmoding of marriage? That is why our girls, in an era in which women are becoming more and more the equals of men (equal, but oh so different!), should receive all possible encouragement to advance towards maturity with a balanced, logical, natural and, above all wholesome attitude towards an instinct second only to that of self-preservation, that of the reproduction of the species.

## 6

## MENSTRUAL FAILURE

A few years ago there was published in *Here's Health* an article I wrote containing the case histories of three young women under treatment for menstrual failure, all of whom recovered about the same time. It was a coincidence which seemed worth reporting and this is still true now that it has happened again. Like many of us I am intrigued both with coincidences and with trinities. At the same time the subject is one of great importance. The implications for a normal, otherwise healthy, and forward-looking young woman of failure to menstruate are very serious indeed and liable to give rise to profound anxiety and depression, particularly in those who are married and anxious to have a baby.

There appear to be no statistics to show us whether this gynaecological phenomenon is on the increase at the present time or not but my impression is that it is far more common than one would expect. I hear of these cases, not only from those actually affected, but from women who attend for the treatment of other ailments and in the course of conversation tell me about others among their acquaintances.

Many who have the ailment go to their doctor for treatment, and unfortunately many of the latter, without the slightest hesitation, will prescribe the contraceptive pill. This, in addition to serving its original purpose, has become a sort of gynae-cological cure-all in the eyes of some doctors who, being busy people, now that we have what is sometimes nicknamed the National *Ill-health* Service, are glad to have an easy way of administering synthetic hormones. Why so many women should be suffering from hormone imbalance is a mystery unless we can blame the pollution of the environment!

The snags which all-too-often arise when the Pill, or hormones in some other form, are prescribed for the treatment of amenorrhoea, is that it gives rise to side-effects which the patient cannot tolerate, but as soon as the drug is withdrawn menstruation ceases and the patient is back to where she started. Clearly something more than the correction of hormone imbalance is required.

## A Year's Menstrual Failure

In July last year Mrs Cartwright came into my London consulting room. My investigation disclosed that she was twenty-two years of age and had been married for three years. Both she and her husband were exceeedingly anxious that she should have a baby but, unfortunately, she had not menstruated for a whole year.

Previous to marriage her menstruation had been normal but on getting married she unwisely, as it turned out, adopted the Pill as a means of contraception, not wanting to conceive during the first year of her marriage. From the start the Pill disagreed with her. Her menstruation became extremely erratic and at times painful and finally stopped altogether about a year before her present visit.

The treatment which I normally employ, and which will be described later, was at once commenced. Since coming to see me involved over an hour's journey I only attended to her at four-weekly intervals, sending her remedies by post in the interval when this was necessary. She turned out to be a very good patient, conscientious, co-operative and appreciative. Her general health improved steadily and she was able to report a marked improvement in her physical relationship with her husband. At my request she kept a fertility chart which, as time went on, began to show increasing indications of ovarian activity. It should be explained here that in constructing a fertility chart a special thermometer, more sensitive than an ordinary one, is used to determine the body temperature at a fixed time just before rising in the morning. This is usually below the recognized figure of 98.6F. When a woman is menstruating normally her early-morning temperature will be lower during the first half of the menstrual cycle than it is in the second half, though the difference may only be a fraction of a degree. Each morning the temperature is recorded on a chart and from this a graph is formed. At the time of ovulation, normally taking place about the fourteenth day after the commencement of the previous menstruation, there will be first a fall and then an appreciable rise in temperature, which will be indicated by a peak in the graph.

When treating a woman for amenorrhoea and infertility it is important that the practitioner should know whether his patient is ovulating or not. When I studied the chart during Mrs Cartwright's visit in November I was encouraged to note a distinct peak about two days previously. On 3rd December she rang me up in great excitement to inform me a period had begun — the first for eighteen months. I learned subsequently that it lasted four days, was normal in amount and there was little or no pain. The remarkable thing about this particular case is that when the patient visited me, roughly six weeks after the resumption of menstruation, I discovered she was pregnant. There had been no further menstruation. It would appear that on or about 19th November Mrs Cartwright not only ovulated for the first time for more than a year but she also conceived. Another valid assumption is that her husband's fertility is of a high order. Apart from nausea during the first few weeks the pregnancy progressed in a satisfactory manner and in due course she gave birth to a healthy baby girl.

Success was achieved in a shorter time in the case of Mrs Harmsworth, who first visited me in August 1972.

### Erratic Periods

From the age of fourteen-and-a-half, when she first menstruated, her periods had always been erratic, often with lengthy intervals between them. She married at the age of twenty-two, some two-and-a-half years before her visit to me. Shortly before her marriage she sought medical advice and was prescribed the contraceptive pill by a gynaecologist. Although she did not feel happy about this form of therapy it did, in fact, bring about greater regularity, although the loss was too heavy to be comfortable and there were other objections, especially loss of sexual feeling and an unwelcome increase in weight. Wishing to have a baby she gave up the Pill about a year before seeing me, when regular menstruation promptly stopped once again.

I at once instituted the usual treatment, consisting of the prescription of supplementary nutrients and homoeopathic and herbal medicines and occasional sessions for osteopathic manipulation. She too was instructed to keep a temperature chart. When she had been attending me for six months she phoned one morning to report that she had had a completely normal menstrual period lasting five days and with an absence of discomfort. Since then menstruation has been regular and we hope it will not be long before conception, which both she and her husband desire, will come about.

## Dieting Stopped Periods

The third case I shall describe is that of Miss Barber, a charming girl of seventeen. Prior to her visit her mother thoughtfully wrote me a most useful case history. Her childhood was normal and healthy in every way and she started menstruation at the age of twelve. This continued to be regular until she was fourteen, at which age she became over-conscious of her figure. In order to reduce weight she starved herself to such an extent that, to use her mother's words, 'she looked like something out of Belsen'. Her periods stopped and her hair fell out. This, alas, is all-too-common a happening with young girls and the most regrettable thing about it is that once menstruation ceases it is very difficult to get it started again. Miss Barber proved to be a very conscientious and co-operative patient, attending me regularly and taking the remedies prescribed exactly as directed. We had many discussions about her problem and other matters with which youth of today is much concerned. Like most of my patients she had sane and wholesome ideas about love and marriage and was not at all in tune with what we have come to call 'permissiveness'.

Perhaps it was a reward for her conscientiousness that after no more than six months' treatment she phoned to give me the good news that for the first time in three years she had a normal menstruation.

As already noted, the most common cause of amenorrhoea in girls and young women is injudicious dieting. It has further been noted that in the majority of cases the response to estrogen, whether it be administered separately as a drug or in combination with progesterone in the form of the contraceptive pill, is usually a positive one. Menstruation will recommence but stops as soon as the remedy is withdrawn. Most patients in such a position give up this form of treatment, either because they do not wish to become dependent on the drug, fearing it might seriously damage their health in other respects, or because there were alarming side-effects such as bleeding between periods, periods which become heavy and prolonged or tendency to gain weight rapidly. From these observations it is quite clear that the disorder is basically one of hormone imbalance and that in many cases this is brought about by nutritional deficiency. There must be elements in the foods we eat that act as precursors of estrogen. An example of a precursor common in a vegetarian diet is carotene, which by means of biochemical action after consumption is converted into vitamin A.

We are becoming increasingly aware, now that herbal medicine is returning to its rightful position in the therapeutic armamentarium and replacing synthetic drugs among those of us who value our basic well-being, that medicinal herbs contain an immense variety of vital substances hitherto unsuspected. Recent research has shown this to be the case and provides a strong reason for an acceleration of research. Herbal medicine having received the seal of official approval through its recognition in the Medicines Act of 1969, it has become an urgent necessity for the National Institute of Medical Herbalists to establish a research centre. As matters are at present a great many of our most valuable herbal medicines have what may be called an empirical status. (Empiricism means skill or knowledge based on experience and not on proof arrived at through controlled trial). It is the empirical aspect of medical herbalism which puts us at a disadvantage with the medical profession, which refuses to accept any form of therapy without positive proof of its efficacy demonstrated by trial involving a large number of patients. Fortunately this supposed weakness in medical herbalism, as seen by the medical profession, has not prevented its acceptance under the terms of the Medicines Act, but the time has come when we ought to begin the proving of our remedies and for this we need a research centre.

### Treating Amenorrhoea

Among herbal medicines there are many which are classified as 'emmenagogues', meaning remedies which induce menstruation. There can be little doubt that an analytical investigation of these medicines, of the kind that could be carried out if we had a research centre, would disclose the presence of estrogen, or precursors of estrogen, and possibly other hormones of gynaecological significance as well. The herbal remedies from which I have achieved most success in treating amenorrhoea include *Agnus Castus, Chamaelirium luteum, Aletris farinosa* and the familiar *Liquorice*.

In the treatment of menstrual failure there is much else to be done besides prescribing suitable herbal remedies. Considering that so many girls cease to menstruate as a result of injudicious dieting, immediate steps must be taken to restore optimum nutrition. The diet should be high in protein and vitamins and relatively low in carbohydrates and fats. It will almost certainly be necessary to prescribe supplementary nutrients, which include minerals as well as all five important vitamins in correct proportion. Regular exercise in the open air is most advisable. In the event of the patient being overweight the diet must be organized with a view to bringing about a reduction to normal.

Psychotherapy plays an important role in the treatment of all types of amenorrhoea, but it is particularly applicable to those which appear to be psychogenic in origin. A variable amount of anxiety and emotional tension is likely in all women and girls whose menstruation is unduly delayed. The anxiety may either be the cause of the amenorrhoea or be caused by it. In either case a sympathetic and understanding attitude on the part of the practitioner, as it relates to the patient's emotional and sexual behaviour, will accomplish a great deal towards relieving the disorder and the anxiety. The young patient must be given the opportunity to ventilate her feelings and fantasies regarding menstruation, sex problems and childbearing. This may enable the practitioner to clear up any misconceptions which the patient entertains on these subjects. Although we live in times in which sex matters are much more freely discussed than used to be the case, and the subject is now taught in schools in a more realistic fashion than some parents care for, it is surprising how much ignorance of basic principles still exist and how strong are the inhibitions in some cases. Unreasonable inhibitions concerning aspects of sexual impulses and reactions which are, in fact, quite normal, must be gradually broken down both by explanation and by discussion if the patient can be persuaded to talk freely, as is much to be desired.

Two of the young women whose case histories have been described in this chapter were in the early twenties but the problem of menstrual failure most often begins to arise when girls are aged between fifteen and seventeen. Although some girls reach this age without ever menstruating, it happens far more often that they begin to menstruate between the ages of twelve and fourteen, continue to do so fairly normally for a year or two, and then come to a sudden stop.

Mothers should realize in these circumstances that their daughters are more likely to respond to treatment without unduly prolonged attendance upon a practitioner, if valuable time is not lost. The condition is more likely to become chronic the longer it is allowed to persist.

## 7

# GETTING MARRIED

One of our most basic needs as human beings is to love and be loved. We need to be accepted as persons, as whole persons, for what we are, for our own sakes. And we need to give ourselves, if we are to find fulfilment, to others and for others, for their own sakes. This is what real love means. It is the basis of everything else that matters, security, happiness and a sense of purpose.

I have said this about the meaning of life as a whole because it is only in this setting that I can speak of the meaning of marriage, for marriage is the most intimate way in which we fulfil this basic need of our lives, to love and be loved, to be accepted and to give with the whole of our being. It is also the reason why those getting married so often feel themselves closer to the heart and meaning of life than ever before.

The purpose of this introduction is to make clear what, in my view, the spiritual ingredients of a marriage should be if it is to have a good chance of being successful, from the point of view of both parties, and enduring. As a gynaecologist I am, of course, concerned more with the physical content of a marriage than the spiritual but I recognize that the two components are at least equal in importance.

In this age of permissiveness there will, in many cases, have been at least a degree of experimentation with what constitutes the physical, or more precisely, the sexual part of a marriage and it must be hoped that this will not have led to a forced marriage in which the all-important ingredients of mutual respect and spiritual affinity, as defined in my opening paragraphs, are lacking.

There are among us many who urge strongly and persistently that there should be more sexual freedom — even among school children — but it is very doubtful if in the long run this will result in a community in which there is more contentment with life, more social stability and more security for the children we produce.

Many of the objects of those who call themselves humanists are admirable but it is worth noting that although they seek the secularization of all ceremonies, including that of marriage, one can find in their literature nothing tangible to replace the stabilizing influence of the Christian code of ethics.

In a world where we see so many things which have endured for centuries being changed solely for the sake of change, it would seem there is consolation in the fact that so far the institution of marriage is not under attack to any extent. A writer who appears to wear the humanist label is worth quoting: 'I am a very strong believer in marriage, and even if I were not it is still a hard fact that more than 90 per cent of people get married.'

## Teenage Marriages

At the present time there is a tendency in all levels of society for couples to marry at an earlier age than used to be the case. Marriages where both partners are still in their teens are becoming common. We are able to perform the physical functions associated with reproduction as soon as puberty is reached at the average age of fourteen or fifteen, but I am sure that marriage at such an early age is highly undesirable for a variety of reasons.

Although puberty comes much earlier, the age of physical maturity in women is from twenty to twenty-five and in men some five years later. At the age of twenty to twenty-five a woman has the lowest risk of being infertile, the greatest likelihood of having strong and healthy children, the lowest risk of having a miscarriage or bringing forth a baby that is physically or mentally defective.

When couples who embark upon marriage have scarcely completed their basic education, have not had time to acquire a proper sense of proportion and of responsibility, nor time to save money, but are almost entirely dependent on their parents or the hire-purchase system for the means of setting up a home of their own, do they not approach marriage far too lightly and thus belittle it?

Since we have long departed from the patriarchal system I am sure they do. The existence of the welfare state confers many benefits, but I do not think making teenage marriages possible is one of them.

I do not have statistics for this country but those from the United States are significant enough. Where both bride and groom are teenagers, 54 per cent of marriages end in divorce. When only the bride is a teenager, the divorce rate is 36 per cent. When both are twenty years of age or over the divorce percentage is 18 only — but bad enough.

When we consider the opposite extreme, that is late marriages, either in the last decade of productive life, or at the time of the menopause in the woman, professional advice should almost certainly be sought when such a marriage is contemplated. In the former, the possibility of child-bearing has to be considered and the physical fitness of the woman for this determined.

At the time of the menopause marriage should be postponed when irregular bleeding persists, because in such circumstances severe haemorrhage can result from sexual congress. In any case, a physical examination is necessary to exclude the possibility of there being some genital disease that might be aggravated by marital relations, or any other morbid condition that might be made worse in the same way.

Considerable discrepancy in age need not necessarily be a disadvantage, provided the man is the elder party. When the discrepancy is in the other direction, serious difficulties are liable to arise when the woman reaches the change of life. In all cases it is as well that the husband should be a year or two older than his wife.

### Choice of a Mate

Books have been written about the complex and baffling subject of the choice of a mate, so I shall not be expected to offer a solution for this problem in a few sentences. However, when a couple are obviously well-mated they are not only a joy to themselves and the children they may have, but to all who come into contact with them, so this ideal is well worth striving for.

Needless to say, hasty marriages are almost always a mistake and we have already concluded that teenage marriages are best avoided. It is better that both should have reached years of greater discretion and have had a number of preliminary contacts. Perhaps incompatibility of temperament is the greatest enemy of harmony, for there is nothing that makes greater demands on tolerance, unselfishness, forgiveness and thoughtfulness on the part of both partners than marriage.

When there is competition to dominate, most men will feel resentful and deprived of their traditional role. My conclusion, from having had the confidence of countless wives in the course of my practice, is that those who have no difficulty in accepting the dominant role in their husbands are happiest. Perhaps I should say dominant in his own sphere, because any sensible husband will appreciate that there are matters over which his wife must have undisputed control. What these are will vary in different cases and must be worked out in the process of adjustment.

To have a clearly recognized division of responsibilities for both partners is a great asset. It might be said that in cases where this comes about, a reversal of the traditional roles is more likely to be harmonious than one in which neither has a recognized role.

I have noticed that almost all women dislike a selfish man. I am sure mutual respect will do more than anything to ensure the happiness and stability of a marriage. It is this that can be relied upon to bring about that deep and lasting affection which should replace the earlier years of ardent and passionate love of which vivid and intensely moving descriptions can be read in prose and verse in every language.

## Honeymoon Difficulties

Under ordinary conditions much nervous excitement is commonly experienced as the date fixed for the marriage draws near. There are all kinds of arrangements to be organized, duties to be performed and visits to be made, all this culminating in the final excitement of the wedding day. When on top of the excitement is super-added a fatiguing honeymoon embracing everything except rest and quietness, it is not surprising that the first weeks of marriage are all too often clouded by unexpected disharmony, the result of jaded nerves.

The need for a restful honeymoon is the greater because through normal sexual union the reproductive system is incited into unaccustomed activity and this activity implies stimulation of the nervous system, of the endocrine glands and of the sexual organs themselves. Both before and after the wedding the menstrual period, which might formerly have been regular, is liable to be upset and commence too early or too late. This is not a serious matter unless it persists but if it does it would be advisable to consult a practitioner about it.

Excessive sexual activity, liable to occur during the honeymoon, quite often results in severe irritation in the vulva and urethra of the wife. So common indeed is this disorder that it has been named 'honeymoon cystitis'. The treatment is to cease indulgence for a few days and apply a soothing ointment, such as chickweed, to the area. If the wife has had a pre-marital consultation her practitioner, if he is thoughtful, will have provided her with this and a further remedy to take internally as a precaution.

It often happens, turning to the bright side, that women who have previously suffered from painful menstruation become better after marriage. This remark should not, however, be taken to mean that this kind of derangement can be left untreated in anticipation of marriage. Such neglect is risky and could lead to chronic ill-health.

Nothing I have written about the physical and mental strains apt to arise in the early days must be held to detract from the great value of marriage to a woman. When happily married, her outlook on life is completely altered. Her surroundings and the making of a happy home stimulate her and she blossoms and matures. Although most young married women now work outside the home, there is a natural desire in almost every normal woman to have children and devote herself exclusively to these and to her husband and her home. I must hasten to add that in all this the husband must play his part enthusiastically. Responsibility for the success of a marriage rests equally upon both partners.

### Pre-Marital Consultation

I recommend strongly that both partners, but the woman in particular, should have a pre-marital consultation with a reliable and experienced practitioner. A great many who have been to see me several months *after* the wedding would have been saved much perplexity, mental strain and acute unhappiness if they had come before the ceremony.

I am sure a lot of what we read in the popular press and in magazines about sexual activity indulged in before marriage, in which it is made to appear that this is now the rule rather than the exception, is exaggerated and intended to be sensational. I appreciate that during serious courtship the strain of remaining celibate may be great enough to bring about a severe conflict of conscience. We must bear in mind that in the young the sexual urge can be very strong indeed and view the matter with sympathetic understanding.

It is in this situation that a consultation with an understanding practitioner can be helpful. The important subject of contraception will be particularly relevant and the various methods available can be reviewed. It can be pointed out that if there must be pre-marital relations then the possibility of an unwanted pregnancy should be guarded against as effectively as possible.

The opportunity will be taken by any right-minded practitioner to warn his young patient against the temptation to become a convert to the contraceptive pill. Those who regularly read my articles in *Here's Health* will be aware that I regard the pill with much disfavour, believing it to be a great menace to gynaecological health and, in the long run, to the general well-being of a woman. There are a number of other forms of contraception which are safe and do not involve any risk to health.

When considering the matter of a pre-marital consultation, it will surprise the sophisticated to know that the practitioner often has to explain to the young man, as well as to the young woman, some of the facts of life that most of us assume are learned in adolescence, if not before. Much more often it is the refinements of the physical relationship regarding which there is ignorance, but it is these very refinements that go far to enhance the enjoyment of the physical content of the union.

There can be no question that the pre-marital consultation must include a complete physical examination, with emphasis on the gynaecological situation in the case of the woman. It is a regrettable fact that quite a number of women who come to see me about problems that arise after marriage do so because after months, or even years, the union has not been physically consummated. Occasionally the fault lies with the husband, but more often it is with the wife. The problem may be either physical or psychological in origin but most often it is psychosomatic, which means a combination of both.

## 8

## PLANNING THE HEALTHY BABY

To many of us not directly involved, the thalidomide disaster will now be nothing but a memory. With the parents and the victims themselves it is a very different matter and they are numbered in thousands.

This drug, responsible for so much unhappiness and distress, and such an upheaval of family life in so many homes, was invented in Germany by the pharmaceutical firm of Gruenthals, given the name Contergan, and first became available in 1961 in Germany. Subsequently it was manufactured in Britain under licence and distributed by the Distillers Company as Thalidomide.

The drug quickly became popular as a tranquillizer and was freely prescribed for the purpose of inducing a comfortable night's rest. It was, as it happened, particularly popular with pregnant women. Alas! When the time came for these women to deliver their babies they found to their horror and dismay that the infants were grossly deformed. Many were entirely without limbs, whilst others only had stumps where their limbs ought to have been. The drug was withdrawn as soon as its evil effect was recognized, but not until something like 5,000 deformed babies had been born alive in Germany alone. In Britain, where the drug was not introduced until a good deal later than in Germany, there are said to be about 350 children who have survived to this day, whilst in Germany about 2,000 are still alive. The victims are now nearing the age of puberty and this is giving rise to social problems. Psychologists are debating whether they should be segregated from the community or integrated with it, or whether they should go to special schools.

Needless to say, the thalidomide affair caused a revolution in pharmaceutical practice throughout the world. In most countries governments, in consultation with industry, got down to the business of amending the laws and practices of pharmacy, to prevent, as far as possible, any repetition of the tragedy.

**The Dunlop Committee**
The result in Britain was to bring into being the Dunlop

Committee, which now exercises an effective control over both the introduction and the sale of drugs. The pharmaceutical industry has organized an intermediate stage between testing on animals and general human volunteers. Even when a preparation has been generally released the Committee continues to exercise a monitoring function. Doctors are enjoined to report to it any untoward side-effects. It now takes from five to seven years for a new drug to reach the market in Britain but when thalidomide first came upon the scene the whole process of testing could be completed in a few months.

In retrospect, perhaps we can say that the only good thing about the thalidomide disaster is that it alerted the whole world in a most dramatic fashion to the potential risk pregnant women run of endangering the well-being of their baby if they take any drug at all. It is now recognized that no drug can be written off as harmless. Many a reputation for innocence has been destroyed in the last few years, and not least the reputation of the ubiquitous aspirin. There is mounting evidence of the serious complications it can produce.

Another result of the thalidomide tragedy was the enactment by our Parliament of the Medicines Act in 1968. Regulations drawn up with the authority of the Act have given the force of law to what was formerly a voluntary system of drug control. A gratifying result of the discussions which took place in Parliament, whilst the Medicines Act was in the committee stage, was a recognition of the virtues of herbal medicine. The practice of medical herbalism is legalized in the Act and we now know that almost all herbal remedies in common use have been accepted as safe by the Dunlop Committee.

I have introduced this chapter with an account of the thalidomide affair, not to harass the minds of mothers-to-be, but for the opposite reason of giving them confidence that no such drug is now likely to come their way, either by accident or design.

Nevertheless, there are still many parents expecting their first-born who are filled with anxiety in case it should turn out not to be normal in every way.

I must hasten to assure these over-anxious parents that the possibility of such a misfortune happening is very remote, especially when it is likely to be the case that the mother-to-be at any rate is doing her best to follow a wholesome way of life in common with most of those who will read this book.

## Hereditary Diseases

When a couple contemplate marriage they ought to give thought to their respective backgrounds, taking into consideration the fact that some diseases can be transmitted from parents to their children. A few examples will be given.

About one third of all cases of epilepsy occur in families subject to this disorder; whilst out of ten children of epileptics, one is likely to develop the ailment.

Among mental disorders, manic-depressive insanity and schizophrenia have a tendency to appear in children of parents afflicted in these ways, and like the majority of mental conditions, and physical ailments also for that matter, are apt to be most pronounced in children of whom both parents are afflicted.

Other ailments liable to be transmitted from parents to their children are coronary artery disease, high blood-pressure, diabetes, skin diseases, asthma and hay fever, rheumatism, colour-blindness, cataract and deafness.

Since it is well known that inherited disadvantages, if they are not too serious, can be to a great extent counterbalanced by environment, prospective parents, in the knowledge that they will do all in their power to provide a wholesome environment for their offspring when they come, should not be unduly worried by these hereditary implications, with one exception: if there has been one of the mental disorders mentioned in both their families, a couple would not be justified in getting married unless they were fully resolved to forego the privilege of having children. I would go so far as to say there would be a strong case here for the sterilization of one or other of the partners.

## Hazards to Foetus

A number of viruses causing infection in the mother can be transmitted to her foetus. Of these, German measles is the most important. It can cause deafness and blindness as well as damage to the developing brain and heart. The foetus is at risk up to the ninth or tenth week of pregnancy and during this period it is of the utmost importance that the mother-to-be should avoid any contact with a case of German measles. Vaccination against German measles is now available for girls aged from ten to thirteen but a decision whether the service should be taken advantage of or not must rest with the parents. With so many injections and vaccines now being offered to children, many parents are seriously concerned lest the remedies should prove to be worse, in the long run, than the ailments they seek to prevent.

X-rays can have a damaging effect on the foetus and should not be resorted to, especially prior to the third or fourth month of pregnancy. There is increasing evidence that obstetric radiography is liable to cause the development of cancer in children.

It is not only the more potent drugs that must be avoided by pregnant women. The familiar aspirin has been under attack in the medical press of late for a variety of reasons and one of the latest to be stated is that its ingestion may increase the likelihood of congenital defects.

Scientists at the Population Genetics Unit at Oxford have stated recently that there is a risk of deformity in children subsequently born to women who have been undergoing treatment for a chronic rheumatic disease with a drug called *Phenylbutazone*.

One of the most common drugs used to treat diarrhoea has been freely available without prescription in Britain since 1935. The drug is *Clioquinol*, better known by the trade-name 'Entero-Vioform'. This drug is now suspected of being the cause of a serious disorder of the nervous system known as 'smon' and has been totally banned in Japan. The possibility cannot be excluded that taking the drug by the mother-to-be could endanger the foetus.

A team of research workers in Stockholm have been studying the possible effect on the foetus in the event of the mother having had cortisone treatment. Animal experiments suggest that cortisone can adversely affect the cellular fluid of unfertilized ova in such a way that in the event of one of the ova being fertilized, bringing about conception, there could be a birth defect. The one most likely to occur in these circumstances would be cleft palate.

One of the commonest disorders of new-born babies is pyloric stenosis. In this condition a thickening of the muscular outlet of the stomach leads to vomiting of feeds in the first few days or weeks of life. Experiments have shown that this disorder is much more common in babies whose mothers have, for some reason or other, been over-anxious during their pregnancy and as a result have suffered from what is commonly known as a 'nervous stomach'. Such a condition is believed to cause the hormone, gastrin, to cross the placenta and enter the unborn baby's blood stream. The effect of this will be to cause the baby to be more liable to suffer from vomiting in its early life than would otherwise be the case.

## Breast Milk Jaundice

The contraceptive pill, with good reason, is held responsible for a variety of disorders in women who make use of it. It is now thought to be the explanation for a form of jaundice affecting babies in early life. Several reports have recently appeared showing that this neo-natal jaundice is becoming more common in breast-fed babies than in bottle-fed babies. In an article in the *British Medical Journal* it is reported that mothers of babies with breast milk jaundice frequently used the pill before becoming pregnant. Investigations carried out in the special-care baby unit at Birmingham Maternity Hospital strongly suggest that the pill is to blame for the disorder. The odds against this being a chance finding are said to be 2,000 to one. Among the severely jaundiced babies, fourteen had mothers who had been on the pill and four had not. It is significant that breast milk jaundice was first recorded in 1963, only a year or two after the widespread introduction of the pill.

## The Rhesus Factor

A disease of newborn infants associated with the Rhesus blood factor has the technical name *Erythroblastosis*. A blood factor is a physical substance which some people have in their blood and some do not. If a blood factor gets into the blood of a person who has not inherited it, it acts like a foreign protein and the body creates antibodies that antagonize the factor, much the same as antibiotics against measles viruses are built up to give immunity to measles. But some antibodies do not protect but cause damage.

About 85 per cent of women have the Rh factor and are Rh positive or Rh+. The remainder are Rh negative or Rh-. If an Rh- mother and an Rh+ father conceive a baby, the foetus growing in the uterus produces Rh factor and some of it may pass into the mother's bloodstream. In that case the mother produces an antibody that is hostile to the Rh factor, which to her body is a foreign substance. This antibody may cross back to the baby with destructive action on its red blood cells. The extent of this destruction determines the severity of the Rh disease or *Erythroblastosis.*

Most Rh- women with Rh+ husbands can produce one or two healthy babies or even more. Usually Rh disease does not manifest itself until the third or subsequent pregnancy. The maternal and foetal circulations do not intermingle and it is thought that the back-and-forth transfer of Rh factor disease antibodies may be affected by 'leaks' in minute capillaries.

Blood studies of pregnant women determine their Rh status. If a patient is Rh+ there is nothing to worry about. If she is Rh- and has an Rh+ husband, there might be a complication in an existing or future pregnancy but the odds are favourable. Only about one in twenty will have an affected baby and this does not usually happen until a third or later pregnancy.

There is at present no known way of preventing Rh disease other than to forbid the union of an Rh- woman and Rh+ man, which a devoted couple would hardly contemplate. They ought, however to make a firm decision to limit themselves to two babies. If they are unfortunate and their second baby developed the disease it might not be so severe as to warrant recourse to the only remedy at present available, which is a blood transfusion. It will be obvious that couples contemplating marriage should have their blood tested.

Mechanical factors operating inside the uterus can cause malformations of the baby. The baby can literally be squashed over a period of weeks so that one or more limbs are deformed. This is a common cause of club-feet and is also one factor in the production of dislocation of the hip. To avoid a mishap of this kind the expectant mother should take care not to wear any tight garment in the abdominal region, should avoid constipation and empty the bladder with reasonable frequency.

Dr Jesse Steinfeld, Surgeon General in the United States, says there is increasing evidence that smoking during pregnancy retards foetal growth, decreases the infant birth rate and increases the incidence of prematurity.

Should would-be parents, on reading this tale of woe, be filled with gloomy forebodings? Not at all, for to be forewarned is to be forearmed. If a pregnancy is properly managed the likelihood of giving birth to a baby who is not physically perfect, strong in constitution, and happy in disposition is remote. Mothers-to-be should have this vision in their minds throughout their pregnancy and it will engender and sustain a determination to do all the right things. At the outset she must make up her mind to avoid all drugs if she possibly can. Only a major illness with her life at stake would warrant recourse to drugs as a last resort, and she might then have to have the pregnancy terminated. Ailments of a less serious nature will respond to rest in bed on a light diet, coupled with the administration of a suitable herbal or homoeopathic remedy whose safety has been demonstrated by generations of usage.

### Nutritional Needs

On the positive side nutrition must occupy a major role.

In a Paper on Congenital Malnutrition, which won a first prize, Mr Stewart of the London School of Hygiene and Tropical Medicine, had this to say:

> A child's size,' its strength of bones and its ability to learn depend on the foods the mother eats during pregnancy, as well as the food given to the child after birth.
>
> Research with animals has proved that the young born to mothers suffering from malnourishment show tremors of the limbs, mental retardation and a general proneness to illness.
>
> Evidence also exists showing similar effects to babies born to mothers who have had a protein-calorie deficiency during pregnancy
>
> Measures taken during the war in rationing and 'cutting back' on 'luxury' products, together with increased consumption of highly nutritious foods, improved the health of teeth, cut still-births and ensured the development of strong bones.

The last paragraph is particularly significant, in that it emphasizes the importance to the prospective mother of having a relatively simple diet chosen for its nutritional virtues and not for its richness. There should be an abundance of fruit, salads and vegetables, whilst the consumption of flesh foods should be sparing, due to their tendency to bring about the development of toxins in the system. Adequate protein intake can be obtained from cheese, eggs, wholemeal bread, peas and beans and milk. In cases where cow's milk is not well tolerated or causes catarrh it might be possible to obtain goat's milk, which is more suitable. Another alternative would be to have a milk substitute, which can be obtained from your health food shop. Yogurt, owing to the beneficial change in its composition brought about by bacterial action, should suit the great majority very well.

In these days when we have unrefutable evidence that there can be a marked deficiency in vital substances in our foods, as a result of the contamination of the environment by chemicals, I regard it as imperative for the well-being of herself and her baby that every pregnant mother should have supplementary nutrients throughout, and as long as she is breast-feeding the baby. All the major vitamins from A to D should be represented in the right proportions and should be derived from natural sources.

The inclusion of vitamin E (d'alpha tocopherol) in the balanced course of vitamins is particularly important. Besides aiding the healthy development of the foetus it will go far to ensure that the mother-to-be will not be afflicted with varicose veins which, unhappily, is all too liable to happen otherwise. Unless the parent has adequate reserves of vitamin E her baby, when born, is liable to develop disorders of various kinds including scleroderma, a condition in which the skin becomes hard like leather, causing stiffening of the joints and leading to gradual wasting of muscle.

It should be noted that mother's milk contains five to seven times more vitamin E than cow's milk, whilst colostrum, which precedes the mother's milk at the time of delivery, is particularly rich in it. Surely we must look upon this as a provision of nature not to be disregarded.

Finally, mothers-to-be must watch their weight very carefully. During the first three months there will be little change, but after that weight will increase rapidly if strict attention is not paid to diet, avoiding an excess of carbohydrates. At the time of delivery the mother's weight should not have increased by much over 20 lbs since conception.

The traditional ideal weight of a newly born baby is 7 lbs. If it is much in excess of this a difficult delivery is liable to result. This, in turn, may involve the use of instruments and the baby runs the risk of injury, especially to the head. I will leave the implications of this to the imagination.

In a leading article on the subject of abnormal children, *The Lancet* (13th November 1971) has this to say:

> The child with physical or mental handicaps needs to grow up in a warm family environment. When a doctor or nurse breaks the news of a child's handicap to his parents he or she probably influences the child's acceptance into the family circle. A cold, insensitive interview may easily increase the parents' anxiety and distress and might lead to the rejection of the child. A sympathetic full explanation of the child's condition to both parents should be only the beginning of the help and advice to be offered to them. It seems clear that mothers of handicapped children are much happier with a full and early explanation of the child's prognosis, and they often feel bitter and angry if the diagnosis is not revealed until several months after birth.

Those especially interested in this subject should also read Chapters Eight and Ten.

I always recommend pregnant women in my care to provide themselves with Margaret Brady's excellent book, *Having a Baby Easily* (Thorsons Publishers Limited).

## 9

## THE MOTHER-TO-BE

It is important to emphasize, before going any further, that in all animals, including the human animal, the reproduction of the species, from conception to delivery, is a perfectly natural process.

Pregnancy is not pathological and must not be treated as though it were an illness. When it happens, because the partners involved want it to happen, it should be looked upon as a supreme blessing consummating the union.

The couple may have waited over-long for the miracle to happen and there may have been times when they doubted their fertility. In such cases as these their joy may be tinged with apprehension. How dreadful it would be if the pregnancy came to an untimely end! Both partners will be filled with determination to do everything they can to assist nature to achieve her ultimate purpose.

Ideally, preparation for motherhood should go back a long way. From the age of ten, the ultimate gynaecological health of young girls should receive consideration.

If they were brought by their mothers for a check-up at yearly intervals from ten onwards, many of the later problems, with menstruation for example, might be avoided. It is so much easier and less costly in time and money to set a girl on the right course at an early age, than to have to treat her for painful menstruation, or no menstruation at all, at the age of sixteen.

Faulty posture and the effect upon health of wrong eating habits are what the practitioner would be looking for. Parents who have done their best to deal with these problems themselves, with scant success, will realize that the results can be very different when the guidance comes from a less familiar, and in the girl's mind, perhaps, a more authoritive source.

A further aid to successful motherhood is that of having a pre-marital examination, when the practitioner may find minor defects that can be easily rectified. He can, at the same time, discuss not only the control of conception, but some of the more intimate problems the young bride may feel anxious about.

When the couple have agreed that the time has come to start a family, they will anxiously await the non-appearance of the usual menstrual period. As it is not my purpose in this chapter to discuss infertility, let us assume that conception will not be long delayed when contraceptive measures have been abandoned.

### 'Morning Sickness'

Soon after menstruation has failed to appear, there will be other indications that conception has taken place. That which young wives dread most is nausea and vomiting, commonly known as 'morning sickness'. Nausea may continue with varying intensity for the first three months and then cease abruptly about the time when the woman has missed her third period. It is usually worse at breakfast, may subside in the afternoon and recur in the evening.

Characteristic breast changes which may be noticed are an increase of the size of the pigmented area around the nipple (areola) and the presence of enlarged glands in the same area. The breasts may increase in size and weight so that a larger brassière may be required. This increase also happens in some prior to the onset of a regular menstrual cycle, but the degree of breast change is much greater in pregnancy and is maintained.

About three weeks after the missed period a practitioner will be able to make a diagnosis on pelvic examination. The laboratory test of the urine will confirm the diagnosis in cases when it is particularly important to know whether or not a woman is pregnant.

Women who become pregnant for the first time, and those who have had miscarriages, are strongly advised to seek the aid of a practitioner, who will take care of her. This will ensure that everything is done to maintain the health and well-being of both mother and baby and will also serve to give the former confidence. There is no time when constant care and supervision is more important.

### Dietary Precautions

The first consideration must be the nutrition of the patient, which is of paramount importance. Ideally, the lacto-vegetarian diet is recommended, but in non-vegetarians emphasis in the direction of vegetarianism, and away from flesh foods liable to load the system with toxins, will suffice. In any case foods with a high content of fat, and spicy and highly seasoned foods, must be given up.

The consumption of carbohydrates, particularly white sugar and white bread, must be strictly controlled. Women who are liable to flatulence may find that a vegetarian diet will increase the tendency. This is due to fermentation in the intestines arising from inadequate digestion. The best remedy is to take care that everything is well chewed, especially in the case of salads and other raw foods.

The intake of protein and calcium must be adequate. Non-vegetarians should have a portion of meat, fish or fowl daily, whilst vegetarians can rely on eggs, cheese and the pulses for protein. Milk is a good source of calcium, and up to two pints a day must be taken by women who are not liable to catarrh. A woman is liable to catarrh could have more cheese and eggs, and her practitioner would probably prescribe a supplementary nutrient rich in calcium. There are a number of excellent milk substitutes available in health food shops.

At a time when the quality of our foods is so much reduced as a result of intensive methods of production, contamination with many chemicals and excessive processing, it is extremely difficult to be certain we are adequately nourished by our foods alone.

I am afraid in this day and age, many of us are obliged to resort to supplementary nutrients, and this applies particularly to those who are run down in health, those convalescent after an illness or an operation and, most of all, to the pregnant woman.

Adequate nutrition with her is a most emphatic must and the reward will be great, both for her and for her baby. She will be far less likely to develop the disorders associated with pregnancy, whilst her baby will stand a far better chance of being born with a good constitution and a happy disposition.

## Supplementary Vitamins

When prescribing supplementary vitamins and minerals, whether for a mother-to-be or for a convalescent person, the criteria must be that they are derived from natural sources and are in proper balance. If proportion is not considered and too much is taken of one particular vitamin, and not enough of others, the results will be disappointing. Deficiency symptoms may develop relating to one of the neglected vitamins. Many spend their money unwisely on vitamins because they are unaware of these principles.

Pregnant women who attend National Health clinics are invariably given some form of iron tablet as a matter of routine whether they need it or not. Iron in the form usually given disagrees with many women and is often totally unnecessary. If the blood count is not less than 80 per cent it would be better to rely upon the choice of food and the supplementary nutrients to maintain the blood in good condition.

Should there be definite indications of anaemia, the medical herbalist or naturopathic practitioner will prescribe suitable remedies which might include a form of iron not likely to have unpleasant side-effects. Also some adjustment in diet would be suggested.

Each time the mother-to-be attends for treatment she is weighed. During the first three months there should be little change but after that the increase might be fairly rapid. In a woman of average height — say 5ft 4 in — the permissible maximum increase in weight during the course of the pregnancy would be 24 lb. In taller women a little more might be permitted and in smaller women rather less.

If the weight increase happens to be low, and even as little as 14 lb, there is no need to worry. It is the excessive gain in weight that is a cause for worry and, when it happens, strict control of diet must be enforced, the intake of carbohydrate being cut to a minimum.

One of the results of improper dieting during pregnancy is likely to be the overweight baby. Not only will this cause delivery complications but the baby itself will have a bad start in life if overweight, and may be constitutionally handicapped. The weight of the baby at birth to be aimed at is the traditional one of 7 lb. If it is a pound more or less than this there will be no need to worry.

As I have already said, women who lean towards the unorthodox forms of therapy, and the principles of wholesome living associated therewith, are strongly advised to place themselves under the care of a practitioner as soon as they know themselves to be pregnant, especially if it is for the first time.

The practitioner experienced in this kind of service will, besides advising on diet and nutrition, institute a proper routine of treatment involving visits at two- to four-weekly intervals according to the patient's convenience.

He will teach her a series of simple breathing and pelvic exercises and give her treatment in the form of neuromuscular manipulation. This is an osteopathic technique particularly valuable in pregnancy because it promotes the circulation of the blood and enhances the functioning of the nervous system, which serves all the organs of the body including the reproductive organs. From long experience I can vouch for the value of this type of treatment, which never fails to give good results.

After the initial adjustment to pregnancy, involving nausea and other discomfort, the patients experience a wonderful feeling of well-being and confidence. Delivery, when it comes about, is seldom difficult, whilst the baby is notable for its good temper and the perfection of its physique.

The mothers, having been encouraged to breast-feed their babies, usually do so with little difficulty. They quickly forget the pains of delivery they may have had and give themselves up to the enjoyment of their offspring.

In the course of time they will be surprised to find that, as a result of the treatment they have received, there is an absence of the unsightly stretch marks on the abdomen which their contemporaries, who have not had this benefit, will be complaining about.

Morning sickness, or nausea, which almost always occurs in the first three months of pregnancy, is both tiresome and distressing. A good plan to alleviate the trouble is to have one or two days' abstinence from solid food.

The mother-to-be should begin the day with a cup of diluted fruit juice. During the day she may have hot clear vegetable broth or yeast extract, as she likes. She can also use carrot juice and apple juice whilst fasting, and in fact at all other times.

Constipation must be avoided. When necessary, an enema of plain warm water may be used, or a herbal aperient taken.

A useful home remedy for this, and for that matter, other forms of biliousness, is gentian-root tea. This might be obtained from a health food shop. It is rather bitter but most helpful.

To aid digestion, what is known as a mono-diet can follow the short fast. One day the mother-to-be can subsist entirely on fresh fruit, the next day on well-soaked prunes and then a day on carrots lightly cooked and so on. Throughout the mono-diet regime she may have drinks as on the fast days but not too near the meals.

In the event of the biliousness being very severe, in spite of following the advice of the practitioner in whose care she has placed herself, he should be asked to prescribe a herbal or homoeopathic remedy. She will need a lot of extra rest during this time.

Throughout the pregnancy, smoking ought to be given up and alcohol restricted to light wines, or Guinness, if preferred.

It will be a part of the practitioner's treatment to see to it that the breasts remain healthy and the nipples in particular. If these are small or sunken, their development must be encouraged by gentle manipulation aided by chickweed ointment. This is very soothing and has great healing properties. The treatment will go far to prevent the formation of breast abscesses and cracking, which so often renders it impossible to breast-feed the baby.

### Breast-Feeding

All of us who have the welfare of mothers and babies truly at heart are strongly in favour of breast-feeding. It is most unfortunate that, for some obscure reason, in many hospitals any excuse is seized upon to discourage the practice. In view of this, the mother must be very strong-minded and insist upon performing her proper function. Her reward will be great, both in her own health and happiness, and that of her baby.

In spite of these advantages, and a number of others that could be mentioned, the pregnant woman must have a genuine desire to breast-feed her baby. If for some reason, perhaps psychological, it is going to be a struggle to do so, it might be more upsetting to the baby than serene mealtimes with the bottle.

A disorder liable to be suffered by the mother-to-be in the later stages of pregnancy is known as 'toxaemia of pregnancy'. It is a form of blood poisoning and a condition your practitioner will do his best to protect you from, for the results can be extremely serious.

The causes of this disorder are still not fully understood but hormone imbalance in the placenta is suspected. Blood-pressure will be checked at each visit and urine analysis will be made. Precautionary measures would include a restriction in salt and fluids, recommending easily digestible proteins, checking the vitamin intake and making sure the kidneys are functioning efficiently.

A less serious, and far more common ailment to which pregnant women are prone, especially with their first baby, is the development of varicose veins. To prevent this happening is another reason for regularly attending a practitioner. The treatment he will give you will do much to prevent this painful and disfiguring disorder. The taking of vitamin E, included in the balanced course of vitamins, will also help.

Although your practitioner will take care of you in a personal way throughout your pregnancy, and give you advice and guidance in regard to matters outside his province, he will not, in all probability, be in a position to assist you in your actual delivery.

He will have advised you at an early stage to contact the doctor with whom you are registered, with a view to your attending an ante-natal clinic and ensuring that a place will be booked for you in a hospital should the need arise.

The decision of whether to have the baby at home, in a nursing home, or in hospital, will be a momentous one. Delivery in hospital should not mean a loss of the humanitarian aspects.

Progressive hospitals encourage the father to be present with his wife during delivery in order that they should share this family experience and enable him to give the support to his wife which only a husband can.

There are a few nursing homes run on Nature Cure lines in which maternity cases will be accepted. In some areas it is possible to engage the services of a midwife — who embraces the enlightened principles of the Natural Childbirth Trust — to supervise the delivery at home.

In the event of your practitioner not being able to give you counsel when making this weighty decision about where to have the baby, you should write to the Natural Childbirth Trust, 41a Reeves Mews, London W1, whose representatives will be found most helpful.

## 10

## FEEDING THE UNDER-FIVES

The feeding of children from birth upwards is a matter about which my advice is often asked.

At the outset I cannot let the opportunity pass of once again stressing the great advantage to both mother and baby of breast-feeding, if this is possible. It is most unfortunate that many doctors now actively discourage the time-honoured custom of feeding babies in the manner nature — in her wisdom — intended they should be fed, without giving any adequate reason apart from the questionable one of making life easier for the mother. It all seems to be part of a general desire in the world of today to standardize everything as much as possible, no matter how artificial life becomes thereby. Women should obey their natural instincts and refuse to be bullied into acting contrarywise.

The ability to breast-feed her baby satisfactorily depends to a considerable extent upon how well the mother herself was fed and otherwise cared for during her pregnancy. Fresh air and adequate sleep and health-promoting exercise, as well as careful dieting, not only influence the health and vitality of herself and her baby during the months of pregnancy, and the ease of the birth itself, but her capacity to obey the dictates of nature afterwards.

Whilst carrying her baby the mother-to-be should give up all refined and over-processed foods, including white flour and sugar, and all the many foods, drinks and confectionery containing them. Make use of good quality dairy produce, have plenty of fruit and vegetables, both lightly cooked, and raw salads. Potatoes should be baked in their jackets. Restrict sugar, especially the white variety, but make full use of honey for sweetening and of molasses for its mineral content and as an aperient. Wholemeal bread should be insisted upon. Meat and fish are not essential and many expectant mothers find these are best omitted. Adequate protein can be obtained from the pulses, dairy products, whole grain cereals and nuts.

Nicotine from smoking, and alcohol in any form, are both poisonous to the developing baby and neither are arrested by the placenta, as is the case with most other substances which might harm the child. Alcohol and smoking also tend to make delivery more difficult and retard growth after delivery. As a concession to mothers who are accustomed to having wine, a glass a day of one of the lighter varieties may be permitted but smoking should be given up altogether.

## Supplementary Nutrients

It has been my experience in attending expectant mothers that, as well as the wholesome and nourishing diet that has been mentioned, supplementary nutrients are immensely helpful in an age in which it is so difficult to obtain a really adequate supply of organically grown fruit, vegetables and salads.

In prescribing supplements it is essential that a careful balance be maintained, so that all vitamins from A to E are represented and that they are from natural sources and not synthetic. Minerals, and calcium in particular, must also be represented. The course which I usually prescribe for non-vegetarians each day is as follows:

For vitamins A and D: two halibut liver oil capsules.

For vitamin B-complex and iron: three proteolized liver with added $B_{12}$ capsules.

For vitamin C: three capsules or tablets of rose hip or acerola — each 100 i.u.

For vitamin E: three capsules of 75 i.u. or 100 i.u. of d'alpha tocopherol.

For minerals and to improve balance: three multivitamin/mineral tablets.

These supplements are best taken at the rate of one each at mealtimes, with the exception of A and D which should be taken separately, say, one on rising and one on retiring. Some nutritionists consider these oil-soluble vitamins are assimilated more effectively if taken with food, but on the other hand, water soluble and oil-soluble vitamins do not go well together, although, oddly enough, this does not seem to apply to Vitamin E. Since natural vitamins should be regarded as foods and not as drugs or medicines, I do not think the time of taking very important but they are less likely to be fully beneficial if all are taken at once instead of at intervals during the day.

The course of vitamins which I have described should be commenced as soon as it is established that conception has occurred and continued until delivery. If the baby is breast-fed the course should continue until weaning, when it may be discontinued gradually. Some mothers not able to obtain organically grown food would benefit from taking supplements indefinitely.

**Natural Sources of Iron**
It has become a routine procedure in the National Health Service to give inorganic iron pills to pregnant women, often without bothering to take a blood count. In many women these cause constipation and other disorders, to say nothing of damaging the teeth. It is far better to rely upon natural sources of iron, such as molasses, to add to what is derived from proteolized liver tablets. Some other good sources of iron are bran, soya flour, eggs, peaches, almonds, pulses, and parsley. Specially formulated iron tablets blended with vitamins can be obtained in most health food shops, to be taken in cases where anaemia is established or suspected. Some iron and Vitamin E are antagonistic – they must not be taken together. The daily requirement of Vitamin E can be taken at breakfast time and of iron on going to bed.

Women who are vegetarians can obtain a non-animal form of Vitamin B-complex tablet instead of that derived from liver, and also acceptable forms of Vitamins A and D.

In the event of the mother not being able to breast-feed her baby at all, in spite of the very strong reasons which make this desirable, she will have to make up her mind what kind of artificial feeding she should resort to. There are many proprietary brands of baby food, all of which have their claims to perfection. If it is decided to use one of these, some trials may be necessary because babies, like grown ups, are choosey. A brand that suits one may not suit another. There is a lot to be said for using modified cows' milk, even though its preparation is rather more complicated.

Considering the present difficulty in getting high quality unpasturized farm milk free from penicillin, it would seem best to decide right away to use one of the unsweetened evaporated milks. This milk is completely sterile and owing to the process of evaporation employed is usually in a form easily digestible by the baby. It should be prepared for use as follows:

3 tablespoons of evaporated milk
4½ ozs cooled, boiled water
1½ to 2 level teaspoons honey
½ to 1 teaspoon of cream from top of bottle of milk (begin with ¼ teaspoon and increase as the baby learns to tolerate it)

This is sufficient for one feed but the baby will require five feeds per day at suitable intervals. If desired, the whole quantity required for the day can be made at one time, increasing all quantities given above as necessary. The whole supply for the day should then be divided into five equal parts and each part put into a separate bottle which has been sterilized by boiling. Keep in a cool place, dark and airy, or in the lower part of the refrigerator. In the latter case the feed should be slightly warmed before use. From the added cream the baby should obtain adequate fat and also vitamin A and D but if desired these substances can be added in another form such as Haliborange or Halibut Liver Oil. This practice may be essential in winter but in summer use cream and let the baby enjoy sunshine as much as possible and thereby obtain Vitamin D from the sun's rays. Cows' milk is low in vitamins in winter.

By the time the baby has reached 16lbs in weight the amount of milk consumed per day will have been gradually increased from 20 ozs to 40 ozs. More than this should not be given or the baby will become over-fat and may develop catarrhal trouble. To reduce bulk progressively less water can be added to the mixture after, say, eight months.

When the baby is about a month old it should be introduced to raw juices. Most mothers start with orange juice but blackcurrant, tomato, carrot and grapefruit are also suitable. At first only a few drops of fresh, strained juice should be given in one tablespoon of cool boiled water. By the time the baby is two months old it can be having up to a teaspoon of fresh juice in two tablespoons of water. Juice can be given with a spoon towards evening. It must be given at least half-an-hour before the milk feed or it may make the baby sick. It is also best to give the juice from 2 to 3 hours after the last milk feed or again it may cause the baby to vomit.

### Solid Food
At the age of three months solid food in the form of fruit and vegetable purée may be introduced. These purées can be bought in tins but are best home-made if this is possible. Apples, pears, apricots, tomatoes, carrots, spinach, prunes and suchlike are all suitable. Start gradually with half a teaspoon or less of the strained purée, gradually increasing at the rate of half a teaspoon a week. This food will have a laxative effect and must not be overdone. It will show in the stools but this is of no significance. Unlike juices, purées should be given just before a

milk feed, preferably the early afternoon one. In the course of time this form of solid food may be given before other milk feeds, ringing the changes in variety, for example, apples in the morning, vegetables at mid-day, and prunes or grapes in the evening. Materials for making purées should be finely sieved and all pips and skins removed. No salt or any other additive should be used. It must always be remembered that most mothers over-feed their babies and far more trouble is caused by this custom than by under-feeding.

At from four to six months the baby must be encouraged to chew by offering him crusts of bread or rusks. At first the mother will have to hold the crust whilst the baby does the nibbling, but soon the baby will learn to hold it himself. Chewing at an early age is important for several reasons. The instinct is strong at an early age and must be fostered, otherwise it is liable to be blunted when later on the baby will refuse hard and tough food and only eat mushes. If this happens, valuable exercise for the jaws and the formation of healthy, strong and well-placed teeth will be jeopardized. Chewing will ensure that the first starchy foods that are eaten will be thoroughly insalivated and this important aid to digestion developed at the right time.

To meet the growing biological needs of the baby for vital substances, cereals should be introduced before the age of six months is reached. Suitable preparations in powdered form designed for mixing with the milk feed can be obtained from your health food shop.

A number of systems of baby feeding have been developed by experts on the subject and a highly important principle in the preparation of foods for these systems is that great care is taken to ensure that they are completely free from pesticide residues. These we know to be the greatest hazard to our health in the present age and they are particularly harmful to babies and small children whose growth and development can be seriously affected by substances having a toxic effect upon the enzyme system. For instance, there is a Swiss rice gruel which is highly nutritious and particularly well tolerated, even by infants as early as the first few days after birth. It can be speedily prepared as an additive to the baby's milk feed. Strained vegetables in jars for use from the third month onwards. Carrots with other vegetables, liver and meat suitable from the sixth month onwards.

We also have from Switzerland baby foods prepared from organically grown cereals. The process employed ensures ready acceptance by infants. These foods are claimed to nourish without causing flabbiness. Colic and minor digestive upsets are usually quite unknown when this food is used.

Unfortunately, these excellent baby foods have not caught on as well as could be wished in Britain, with the result that the demand is not always sufficient to warrant a shop keeping them in stock. It is to be hoped that as mothers become more and more health food conscious the demand will increase rapidly, whereupon the problem of keeping stocks in health food shops will be solved.

More recently, and more successfully, has been the introduction in health food shops of baby muesli. (Readers are advised to consult shop managers on the various brands of health foods available for babies). By the time the baby is a year old the bottle feeds, which by then have been reduced to three a day, will be given up and the baby will be encouraged to drink whole milk from a cup. The regime at this age might be somewhat as follows:

| | |
|---|---|
| *On waking:* | A drink of diluted fresh orange juice. |
| *For breakfast:* | A piece of crusty wholemeal bread with butter and honey. One of the mueslis, of which there is now a big variety in health food shops. Milk in a cup. |
| *Mid-morning:* | A drink of diluted prune or apple juice or some vegetable soup. |
| *Mid-day:* | Up to three tablespoons of vegetables such as carrot pulses or greens, the latter well chopped. Some mashed potato which has been baked or steamed in its skin. About this time or a little later, the sieving of vegetables can be given up. Roughage is needed to promote digestion. A piece of buttered wholemeal bread with grated cheese on it or part of a poached egg. Apple either raw, or baked, pear or peach or fruit salad. Fruit purée with custard or junket. Water to drink at end of meal if wanted. |
| *Tea:* | About two tablespoons fresh raw carrot juice. A salad sandwich made with wholemeal bread or a small separate salad and wholemeal bread and butter. A piece of home-made cake or bread and butter with honey. A drink of milk in a cup. |
| *At bed-time:* | A drink of water or diluted fruit or vegetable juice. |

## Meals at age of three years

| | |
|---|---|
| *On waking:* | A drink of diluted fruit juice. |
| *Breakfast:* | Apple, pear, orange, peach or grapes or dried fruit |

soaked and lightly cooked, or muesli. Wholemeal toast and butter with honey or home-made marmalade. Milk or milk and hot water to drink.

*Mid-morning:*    A drink of diluted fruit juice.

*Mid-day meal:*    Small portions of vegetables mashed or chopped and potato with a little butter. Accompany this with grated cheese, poached or scrambled egg, or mashed pulses. Non-vegetarians could introduce small portions of meat or fish at this age but not every day. For second course, fruit salad or fruit purée with junket or baked or steamed custard. Mother can ring the changes. A drink of water if desired.

*Tea:*    Wholemeal bread and butter or sandwich made with vegetarian pâté, or a salad sandwich using tomato, lettuce or mustard and cress. Home-made cake. A drink of milk. A raw apple if desired on going to bed. A drink of diluted fruit juice.

## Meals for older children

*Breakfast:*    Children should be encouraged to have yogurt to which can be added wheat germ and honey to the taste. Using a yogurt obtained at a health food shop as starter, this can easily be freshly made at home with some saving of expense. There are now also many mueslis available from health food shops, whilst wholewheat flakes constitute an excellent breakfast food. A tablespoonful of grated raw carrot can be added to the flakes, as well as milk, if the child likes this. In winter oatmeal porridge with added honey and milk is recommended. A slice of wholemeal bread and butter with honey or home-made marmalade or jam. Children with large appetites can have a lightly boiled egg.

*Mid-day:*    At the mid-day meal there should always be a generous supply of cooked vegetables and a potato, preferably baked in its jacket. For protein savoury dishes with a base of nuts, one of the vegetarian cookery books can be consulted. At your health food shop you will find many excellent tinned savouries and these are always being added to or improved. Non-vegetarians will wish to give their growing children small portions of poultry, meat or fish but this should not be done more than once a day. As a second course it is desirable to introduce fruit in some form whenever possible. There can also be puddings of baked custard, unpolished rice or barley kernels. Children are usually fond of soup and the midday meal can begin with this, especially in winter.

*Tea:*    This is the meal at which children should be encouraged to eat a raw salad throughout the year.

These salads can vary according to season, using lettuce, tomatoes, raw cabbage heart, raw brussels sprouts, broccoli or cauliflower, carrot and beetroot. To the salad can be added grated cheese, milled nuts or egg. Following the salad there can be wholemeal bread and butter or baked potatoes and butter. Finish the meal with home-made cake or biscuits and a drink of milk.

Children should not be encouraged to have tea or coffee. It is best to confine them to milk or milk and hot water or diluted fruit or vegetable juice.

It is regrettable that there should be such an enormous consumption among children of 'squashes' which are almost entirely synthetic in their composition. Among their components are saccharine (coal tar), glucose (made by treating corn starch with acid), and artificial colouring and flavouring. The proportion of natural fruit juice is minute. The long-term effect upon children of all these chemicals could be extremely harmful. It is gratifying that health-food manufacturers have now come to the rescue by providing us with genuine fruit drinks such as Golden Orange, Golden Lemon and Golden Apple. These juices may seem rather expensive initially but they are highly concentrated and one bottle will make about six pints suitable for drinking.

Much reference has been made in this chapter to milk as a food suitable for babies. It must be pointed out, however, that milk is very catarrh-forming and for this reason may not suit some babies. In these cases a milk substitute should be tried

Those especially interested in the nutrition of the expectant mother should also read Chapters Eight and Nine.

## 11

## INFERTILITY AND CHILDLESSNESS

There is much concern among thinking people about what has come to be called the 'population explosion'. If the human race continues to increase and multiply without let or hindrance it is abundantly clear that the end result could be disastrous. Already in India and other eastern countries it is not possible to produce sufficient food locally to feed the population adequately and thus millions of men, women and children are, quite literally, on the verge of starvation. Much is being done to limit reproduction in these regions by means of various forms of birth control combined with a stream of organized propaganda but, so far, the result has not been spectacular.

When we are aware of this situation it seems incongruous that, at the same time, there are among us countless women who have no need of contraceptives because they lack fertility. For those who have the strong maternal instincts normal in women, this can be a tragic and heart-breaking trick of fate The frustration and distress it engenders is all-too-often revealed in letters which I receive.

### Involuntary Infertility

Involuntary infertility, as distinct from infertility resulting from the employment of contraception, may be defined as failure of conception to take place after one or more years of sufficiently frequent and normal sexual intercourse. In considering this problem the male, as well as the female partner, must be taken into account. It would be unreasonable to devote a lot of attention to the treatment of the latter until, by means of a simple test, the fertility of her partner had been established.

After two or three days of abstinence, a semen sample should be obtained in a test tube for examination. The examination can be carried out at any centre of the Family Planning Association. The address of your nearest one can be obtained from the telephone directory. Alternatively, your doctor or practitioner can arrange the test. A normal sperm count contains 40 to 100 million sperm in each cubic centimetre of semen, whilst two to four c.c. or about a teaspoonful, is considered a normal sample.

When there is complete absence of sperm the situation is virtually hopeless but in those instances in which the sperm are of poor quality, or the count is low, further studies are indicated and the possibility of improvement through suitable treatment exists. In the course of my practice, gratifying results have been obtained by building up the vitality of the male patient by the application of nutritional therapy and the administration of suitable herbal and homoeopathic remedies.

## Basal Body Temperature

In the case of the female it is important to establish whether ovulation occurs at regular intervals. This may be determined by keeping a record of the basal body temperature.

During the phase of the menstrual cycle preceding ovulation, when there is normal estrogenic activity, the basic temperature taken with a suitable thermometer on awakening in the morning will be somewhat below normal, varying from 97° to 97.8°F. After ovulation occurs the basal temperature rises by one half to one degree and remains elevated for about fourteen days but in most cases the graph, which should be constructed, will show a distinct peak preceded by a dip on the day on which ovulation actually occurs.

Your practitioner will probably be able to provide you with the right kind of thermometer, more sensitive than the ordinary clinical thermometer, and with special forms on which to construct a graph and record other relevant information. There will also be detailed directions how to make the best use of the thermometer and chart.

Having established that ovulation takes place normally, the next step would be to ensure that both the general and gynaecological health of the patient is in every way satisfactory, and this will be gone into in some detail further on.

## Fallopian Tubes

In the event of conception not occurring, in spite of there being normal ovulation, and in spite of the health of the patient being good in all respects, the question of establishing that the fallopian tubes are open must be given consideration. These are tube-like structures which are attached on each side to the topmost part of the uterus and are the lines of communication between ovary and uterus. The ovum that is discharged from the ovary is taken up by the funnel-like end of the fallopian tube for transport to the uterus.

It is in one or other of the tubes that fertilization of the ovum by the sperm usually takes place. Sperm deposited in the vaginal canal are attracted to the clear, slippery mucus of the cervical canal. The sperms migrate through this mucus and work their way up the uterus into one or other of the tubes. If a female ovum is present in the tube one of the sperms will attach itself to it and fertilization will then have occurred. Subsequently the fertilized egg (ovum) will descend into the uterine cavity to find a nest for itself in the prepared lining of the uterus. Orthodox gynaecologists employ two kinds of test to establish the 'openness' of the fallopian tubes.

The Rubin test is accomplished by what is known as *insufflation* (blowing a gas or powder into a body cavity) with carbon dioxide, to determine whether the gas in the uterus travels through the tubes into the abdominal cavity. This is determined by a measuring device and the fact that gas in the abdominal cavity irritates the diaphragm, (the breathing muscle at the base of the lungs), after the patient sits up. Referred pain at this stage in one or both shoulders is also an accepted sign that the tubes are patent or open.

More common than the Rubin test, and probably more reliable, is *uterosalpingography*. This involves the injection of iodized oil into the uterus, after which X-rays are taken. The uterus and the tubes are outlined and free oil is dispersed into the abdominal cavity. In the event of one or both tubes being blocked the X-ray will show where the blockage has occurred.

### Sims-Hubner Post-Coital Test

Sometimes another test, known as the Sims-Hubner or post-coital test, is carried out. This is to disclose whether there is any incompatability between the partners in respect to sperm reception by the cervical mucus. The couple are instructed to have sexual intercourse during the night before examination, preferably after two or three days' abstinence. A sample of semen deposited in the vagina is examined next morning in a laboratory. As a rule, the sperm found in the vaginal secretions will have become immobile when examined under a microscope, but the sperm found in the mucus of the cervical canal should show good mobility.

Whilst there can be no question of the desirability of having the very simple male test for fertility carried out, it is open to doubt if the test for patency of the tubes in the female should also be undertaken, in view of the fact that it is far less conclusive and, at the same time, is not at all a pleasant experience for the patient.

There can be two reasons for blockage of the tubes; structural malformation or the presence of an excess of mucus. The two operations described may not, in the event of blockage, indicate which of the two causes is responsible. If there is a serious structural defect in both tubes little can be done to restore fertility. Attempts are sometimes made by gynaecologists to unblock the tubes by means of a surgical operation but cases in which success is claimed are very few indeed. Even when there is initial success the formation of adhesions is likely to bring about renewed blockage in a short time.

Since X-rays of the tubes do not necessarily indicate the cause of the blockage we have the situation in which the indications are inconclusive. If an excessive accumulation of mucus is the cause, an initial operation may indicate total blockage in both tubes, whilst a second operation may show one or both to be open.

Because there is reason to believe that blockage is more often due to mucus than to a structural defect, there is a good case for instituting treatment for a few months with the object of reducing excessive mucus in much the same way that would be done when inflammatory conditions of mucous membrane occur elsewhere in the body. Chronic congestion of the nasal and related sinuses is a good example and in this connection it is worth noting that when a woman has a heavy catarrhal cold there is often a corresponding vaginal discharge.

So far I have dwelt in the main with the condition of the fallopian tubes but there are, of course, many other causes of female infertility. Although it may surprise many readers, one quite often, in the course of practice, comes across cases in which couples who have been married for some time have never had complete intercourse. On examination it will, in these cases, be found that the hymen of the woman is still virtually intact, only admitting one examining finger. Sometimes the couple are unaware that they have not achieved complete intercourse, whilst in other cases the woman is afflicted with vaginissmus. Through fear of pain the musculature surrounding the vagina goes into spasm, rendering penetration impossible.

In the first case a short explanation of the mechanics of sexual intercourse, accompanied by stretching of the hymen to make things easy, will quickly rectify matters. I have had several such cases in which pregnancy followed in a few months.

There are other cases in which no proper intercourse has taken place owing to impotence in the man. He either does not have an erection at all or he has a semi-erection with premature ejaculation. In such a case as this treatment must consist of building up the virility of the male by means of nutritional therapy and the administration of suitable herbal or homoeopathic remedies.

**Excessive Intercourse**
A cause of infertility not usually taken into account is excessive intercourse. In newly married couples daily intercourse is not uncommon and will do no harm, but if frequency is greater than this a condition known as 'azoospermia' may result. This means a pathological lowering of the sperm count in the semen. As a rule, couples practise contraception during the first year or two of marriage, whilst they settle down. When they decide to try for a baby it would be as well to restrict intercourse to twice weekly, except at mid-period times, when it should be more frequent, bearing in mind that in women the time of maximum fertility is from the twelfth to sixteenth day inclusive, counting from the commencement of menstruation in a twenty-eight day cycle.

Other causes of infertility, of which space will not permit a detailed account, are a variety of gynaecological disorders including leucorrhoea, abnormality of the vaginal secretions, malposition of the uterus, inadequate nutrition, smoking, the taking of drugs, obesity and hormone imbalance.

At the commencement of treatment of a case of infertility in a couple, the fertility of the male must first be established. If this is in doubt he must be treated separately.

When the woman comes for a consultation she must be questioned about her menstruation, as to regularity, duration, amount of loss, and whether she has pain at or between periods. The presence of leucorrhoea must be noted and when it commenced. If she has conceived and miscarried, details of the miscarriage which ended the pregnancy should be ascertained. The past medical history, age at marriage, how long married, any family or constitutional disease, are all questions that may throw light upon the problem. There should be an enquiry into sexual intercourse; whether accompanied by pain, pleasure or desire and if it has, in fact, occurred at all. The question of frequency is very important. Finally, the kind of contraception, if any, must be enquired into, bearing in mind that the contraceptive pill is a common cause of infertility as well as gynaecological derangement, whilst any form of contraception employed for an overlengthy period will reduce fertility.

Before any medication is prescribed to promote the fertility of either partner one must be certain that their nutrition is fully adequate. It will usually be found that various supplementary nutrients have been taken intermittently and with little regard to balance and to economy. Almost always I find that a carefully considered balanced course of vitamins and minerals will materially help the situation. Of course, apart from supplements, it is essential that the dietary should also be well-balanced and wholesome. What we call a food reform diet must be introduced if it is not followed already.

## Malposition of Uterus

In the event of there being malposition of the uterus, suitable treatment must be given to correct the disorder. This, as well as employing a special form of gynaecological osteopathy, will consist of learning pelvic exercises. These, together with breathing exercises, will also promote circulation, particularly in the reproductive region where it is most needed in the circumstances. The functioning of the nervous system activating all organs of the body, including the organs of reproduction, will be greatly enhanced by making use of a special form of osteopathy known as neuromuscular manipulation. I always employ this when treating a woman patient for infertility if she is able to attend.

If there is reason to believe that the hormone balance of the patient is not as it should be, we have available a number of herbal remedies which, without being hormones in themselves, have the capacity of stimulating the glands concerned and, in particular, the pituitary gland, to bring about the production of hormones in the right amounts and at the right time in the menstrual cycle.

## Hormones: Regrettable Results

The prescription of hormones, mostly of synthetic origin, by the medical profession to promote fertility, is acknowledged by doctors themselves to be a very dubious procedure and one liable to have regrettable results. I am sure most readers are appalled, as I am, when we read of women who have been given a special form of hormone treatment having multiple births, bearing children in a manner reminiscent of litters of animals. Fifteen is the highest number yet recorded, and this occurred in a Roman housewife. The foetuses, ten female and five male, when removed from the womb, were perfectly formed, measuring about five inches long and weighing just under 5 oz each. The woman was in her fourth month of pregnancy after undergoing a fertility course of a hormone drug. The foetuses had, apparently, died because the woman's womb was too small to accommodate their continued growth.

In the event of the patient having a proneness to catarrhal colds, this condition must be suitably treated in view of what has been said previously about possible blockage of the fallopian tubes with mucus. Suitable adjustments in the dietary are made and suitable medicines are prescribed.

Of great importance is the health of the vaginal secretions, because if this is not as it should be conditions will be very unfavourable for the viability and mobility of the sperm. The acid/alkaline balance must be in proper adjustment and if it is not suitable, vaginal applications must be prescribed to make it so. Tests can easily be made in the consulting room.

In a final word to the woman who is sad because she is childless, let it be said that whether she has been through the whole gamut of treatment as laid down in the medical textbooks without achieving success, or has had no previous treatment of any kind, this is a case in which medical herbalism and naturopathy are well equipped to provide a remedy.

In my experience, aspects of infertility most often neglected, since it is not the custom of physicians to treat the whole person, are the psychological, the nutritional and the physiological. The last mentioned approach, involving osteopathic gynaecology with manipulative treatment, and exercises, holds great promise since it results in bringing the all-important blood supply to those parts where the need is greatest.

The psychological aspect of infertility can best be appreciated when it is explained that over-anxiety is sometimes found to be the sole cause.

## 12

## CERVICAL SMEAR TEST: ITS IMPLICATIONS

All of us dislike the thought of cancer because there is something evil about it. It can attack us in a secret and insidious manner when we appear to be in the pink of condition and develop without our being aware of it, often over a long period. In spite of millions having been subscribed and spent on cancer research we are still unaware of the cause and are without any definite cure.

There is little doubt that the incidence of cancer of all kinds, and in particular, cancer of the lungs, is increasing at an alarming rate and few who concern themselves with the matter will deny that pollution of the environment, in which should be included self-pollution by smoking, is likely to be the major cause of this alarming development.

There are various names for the disease; malignant tumour, cancer, carcinoma. What are they and how do they differ? The best definition of a tumour is a new growth, or technically a neoplasm. Tumours are classified as benign or malignant. The former does not as a rule endanger life but the latter does.

Gynaecologic cancer is the one with which I am concerned and this is a malignant tumour in any part of the female reproductive system or genital tissue. It has been estimated that 10 per cent of all women are liable to develop some gynaecologic malignancy during their lifetime but in my personal experience as a gynaecologist this is unduly pessimistic. Uterine cancer is divided into two types for practical purposes, depending on its location: cancer of the cervix (the mouth of the womb or that part of the organ that projects into the vagina), and cancer of the body of the womb, which lies within the pelvis. Cervical cancer is much more common than fundal cancer and much easier to detect.

### Secondary Tumours
A cancer may be defined as a group of cells that have got out of control and proliferate at an abnormally rapid rate. Different cancers grow at different rates but the amount of local destruction caused by a malignant tumour is only a part of the

problem. We also have to consider a cancer's known ability to spread to other areas of the body and plant malignant seeds that may grow into secondary tumours. This process of spread is called *metastasis*' and the secondary growths are '*metastasus*'.

The most likely reason why surgical operation for the removal of malignant tumours are often unsuccessful is that infected fragments arising from the operation are carried by the circulation of the blood or the lymph to distant parts of the body, where they initiate new growths. This represents a practical demonstration of the metastatic process. I had a patient under my care for ten years whom I suspected throughout to be afflicted with cancer of the uterus, although this was not actually diagnosed until shortly before she died. She was an intelligent and very thoughtful woman and thus well aware of the metastatic implications. She resolutely refused to enter hospital, where a surgical investigation followed by hysterectomy would almost certainly have been carried out. Perhaps she was right in thinking that had this happened her early demise would have been inevitable. We shall never know. Throughout the long period she was under my care she lived wholesomely on a mainly vegetarian diet augmented by supplementary nutrients sufficient to maintain her vitality and, apart from an occasional vaginal haemorrhage, her health was excellent and trouble free. Many times I urged her to have a second opinion about her condition but she would not do so and her husband, who was older and very fragile, but of the same persuasion, supported her. Looking back I see them as a very interesting, very strong minded, very old-fashioned and very lovable couple.

### Pelvic Anatomy
The behaviour of the most-often encountered gynaecologic tumours of a malignant nature is best understood if one has some knowledge of pelvic anatomy. In the pelvis nature has devised an ingenious structural arrangement to accommodate the uterus, the fallopian tubes and the ovaries. Because these organs lie between the bladder in front and the rectum behind and because these latter organs vary in form depending on the presence or absence of urine or faeces, it is clear that the female organs of reproduction cannot be in a fixed position. Instead, they are suspended between bladder and rectum in a hammock-like fashion from ligaments attached higher up in the pelvic

cavity. In this way the uterus, tubes and ovaries are rendered mobile and free to move up or down as the occasion requires. This arrangement is best appreciated if we consider the requirements of pregnancy, that the uterus must be free to rise as it grows in size until eventually it leaves the pelvic area altogether and enters the abdomen.

The cervix is the small end of the pear-shaped uterus and the part that projects into the vagina. It can, when in a normal position, easily be felt by the examining fingers or seen with the aid of a speculum. The canal which runs through the cervix into the uterine cavity makes this accessible also with the aid of instruments. The ovaries, situated as they are higher up in the pelvis, can only be examined from without which makes their condition less easy to determine by the gynaecologist.

This short essay on the anatomy of the reproductive organs enables us to appreciate that the two most frequently encountered gynaecological cancers, cervical and fundal, are easily accessible, and capable of being diagnosed.

## Cervical Smear Test

In recent years there has been so much publicity in women's magazines and through the distribution of leaflets about the cervical smear test that all readers will have heard of it and many will have had it carried out.

This procedure is sometimes known as the P.A.P. test because it owes its development to a distinguished gynaecologist named Papanicolau. The procedure is to obtain a collection of discarded (exfoliated) cells from just inside the cervical canal. In some clinics quite a performance is made of the matter and the patient subjected to unnecessary discomfort through the employment of a vaginal speculum. An experienced practitioner can pick up the cells on a small swab so easily that the patient is hardly aware that it has been done. The sample of cells is sent in a tube to a laboratory where it is microscopically examined by an expert cytologist who will let the practitioner or gynaecologist have a report on the nature of the cells he has identified. In the great majority of cases no abnormal cells will be found, much to the relief of both practitioner and patient. A matter not usually understood by women is that there are many stages between a negative report and one of outright malignancy; consequently, when they are told the report is not negative they are apt to fear the worst. Unfortunately, the pressure on doctors is so great nowadays that there is seldom time to give a proper explanation of her condition to the patient. The line of least resistance is taken and the patient is referred, willy nilly, to hospital for a further investigation. This usually involves dilation and curettage, commonly known as a D. and C. or a 'scrape'. The operation enables a much larger collection of cells to be obtained for further examination. In the event of a pre-cancerous condition being definitely confirmed by this investigation into the cervical canal and cavity of the uterus, one of two procedures will be considered necessary. If the cervix only is infected a surgical operation known as 'conisation' is carried out. This means that a cone of tissue is cut away from the entrance to the uterus taking with it the whole of the area under suspicion. In the event of the body of the uterus being involved a total hysterectomy would be deemed necessary.

The medical herbalist and naturopath is concerned only with laboratory reports on cervical smears which disclose an unhealthy condition of the cervix and vagina. The matter is outside his province when there are definite indications of incipient carcinoma. The most he could then do would be to fully explain the situation and its implications to the patient and recommend her to the care of a trusted medical acquaintance in the event of her not having registered with a local doctor, as is often the case.

Bearing in mind that the medical profession, as a whole, pays far too little attention to the important matter of building up the patient's general health and vitality before an operation and speeding her return to this desirable condition afterwards, there is one other thing the unorthodox practioner can do for his patient. This is to assist her with advice on diet and on the selection of such vitamins and other vital substances of which she stands in need. In my experience there is much confusion about the taking of these supplementary nutrients. Among those who consult me there are very few at the present time who take no supplements of any kind but there are a great many who make an unwise selection in which there is a lack of balance and a failure to recognize the vital substance they need most. Such patients can often be advised how to get better results at less cost.

I have no doubt at all about the value of the cervical smear test and am of the opinion that all women from the age of thirty onwards should have it done at two yearly intervals, preferably by a practitioner, medical or unorthodox, who can be relied upon to give a full interpretation of the report in a case in which it is not unambiguously negative.

## Additional Information

In the course of taking a cervical smear a great deal of additional information can be obtained as a bonus. This includes the condition of the cervix, the nature of the vaginal secretions and whether or not there is atrophy of the vagina, actual or incipient. The latter condition is regrettably common among women who have passed the menopause and is responsible for much distress and frustration. If discovered in its early stages, suitable treatment can do much to alleviate the disorder and permit a resumption of intercourse. Other disorders which may be discovered whilst taking a smear, and given appropriate treatment before they begin to cause distress to the patient, are erosion of the cervix, *trichomonas vaginalis, candida albicans* and the presence of polyps.

*Trichomonas* and *candida* are, respectively, bacterial and fungoid infections which, if not treated, can cause an unhealthy vaginal discharge, often with intense itching and soreness of the vulva. Suitable early treatment can usually effect a speedy cure but if either condition is neglected and allowed to become chronic it can be very resistant to treatment.

Another useful bonus arising from the taking of a cervical smear and its subsequent examination in a laboratory, is that the patient's hormone balance is clearly indicated in some cases and is then of much value to the practitioner when he has to decide if the gynaecological disorder from which his patient may be suffering is due to an excess or to a deficiency of estrogen.

When it is clear from the laboratory report, supported by the gynaecological manifestations of the patient, that estrogen is secreted in excessive quantities, suitable remedies designed to restore normality can be prescribed. Among these would be a naturally derived form of vitamin E (alpha-tocopherol) in generous dosage. If the patient was suffering from heavy and prolonged menstruation at the same time, as might well be the case, her blood count would almost certainly be low and she would need, in addition, Vitamin B-complex with added $B_{12}$ also in generous dosage. In the event of iron having been also prescribed the patient would be warned not to take vitamin E and the iron preparation at the same hour of the day, because the two substances are antagonistic and would tend to nullify each other. Medical herbalists also have other remedies which indirectly restore the hormone balance by their influence on the pituitary gland.

When, as a result of the laboratory report on the cervical smear, supported by such symptoms as lack of menstruation or early menopausal manifestations, a lack of estrogen is confirmed, there is a temptation to prescribe synthetic forms of estrogen or, alternatively, the natural product derived from the urine of pregnant mares or even the contraceptive pill. The latter expedient, in particular, is very popular with some doctors but there are many who condemn the giving of the pill or any other form of estrogen in such circumstances. There is ample evidence that the long term results can be extremely detrimental to the patient's well-being unless the treatment is very strictly supervised and regulated. A far better alternative is to seek a remedy containing elements, such as enzymes or other precursors, which encourage the body to increase its own production of estrogen. Research workers in medical herbalism are constantly discovering new properties in their materials and may soon have the answer to this requirement, if they do not have it already.

## 13

## WOMEN'S HORMONES

Endocrinology is the science which concerns itself with the function of those glands which secrete into the bloodstream one or more specific chemical compounds known as *hormones*. Hormones are chemical messengers which arouse, or set in motion, action in associated organs.

Let us first consider that part of the brain we call the *hypothalamus*, because it is here that we have the connecting link between the highest level of the brain, the cerebral cortex, and the pituitary gland.

We regard the pituitary as the 'master' gland but, nevertheless, there are both stimulatory and inhibitory agents originating in the hypothalamus which direct pituitary function. For instance, disease or injury in the hypothalamus may give rise to such endocrine disorders as sexual precocity, retarded growth, absence of appetite with gross obesity. Emotional disturbances, anxiety and worry, and even wrong thinking, may upset hypothalamic-pituitary mechanisms.

The young wife over-anxious for pregnancy may cease to menstruate and display symptoms indicative of pregnancy, such as nausea and abdominal swelling, yet not be pregnant. Abnormal obesity may occur in maladjusted girls, menstrual disturbance, often with severe flooding, in women experiencing distressing emotional upheavals, and severe endocrine imbalance in neurotic, over-anxious and weight-conscious girls and young women, which sometimes results in a pathological loss of appetite known as *anorexia nervosa*.

The hypothalamus portion of the brain and the pituitary gland are related both anatomically and functionally. Our thoughts, our hopes and joys, our sorrows and our worries, all profoundly influence the hypothalamus-pituitary partnership.

The pituitary gland is situated in a cavity at the base of the skull which can easily be felt and is divided into anterior and posterior parts. It is the anterior part which secretes the hormones which stimulate distant organs; *somatotrophin*, the growth-stimulating hormone, *adreno-corticotrophin* (A.C.H.T.) which stimulates the adrenal cortex, the thyroid-stimulating

(T.H.S.) and *gonadotrophic* hormones which activate the ovaries in women and the testes in men.

The hormones with which we are chiefly concerned in this chapter are those peculiar to the female. These are the gonadotrophins F.S.H. (follicle stimulating hormone) and L.H. (lutenizing hormone). These are directly concerned with menstruation and with procreation.

### The Ovaries

Having discussed the pituitary gland we must now consider the ovaries. When, as a result of a brain signal on or about the fourteenth day of the average menstrual cycle, the pituitary F.S.H. is transmitted by way of the blood stream to one or other of the ovaries, a follicle or capsule within the ovary is activated. The ovum encased in the follicle begins to ripen and, at the same time, *oestrogen* is secreted. The release of oestrogen into the blood stream prepares the lining of the uterus for the reception of a fertilized ovum, should fusion of ovum and sperm take place as a result of sexual intercourse. The milk-producing glands of the breast are also influenced, causing some women to be more than usually conscious of their breasts in this phase of the menstrual cycle.

As activation of the follicle continues, the supply of F.S.H. will cease and no further ova will ripen to bring about the possibility of a multiple pregnancy. Multiple pregnancies result when the action of the hormone F.S.H. is more prolonged than is usually the case.

Upon the release of an ovum, the follicle which contained it is transformed into a temporary auxiliary gland. It continues to produce oestrogen and also another hormone which we call *progesterone.* Progesterone supplements oestrogen in preparing the lining of the uterus for the implantation of a fertilized ova, should there be one. In the event of fertilization taking place, both oestrogen and progesterone continue to be produced and will inhibit the release of any further ova during pregnancy.

Should conception not take place, the menstrual cycle proceeds normally. The ova-containing follicle begins to disintegrate, the lining of the uterus begins to break down and on the twenty-eight day of the menstrual cycle, on average, is sloughed off to produce the menstrual flow. The cycle then starts all over again.

It has been necessary to explain in detail the processes of the pituitary gland and the ovaries, and the hormones they produce, in order to focus attention upon the immense importance of the two hormones oestrogen and progesterone in the gynaecological well-being of women. Many of the disorders from which women suffer in this area are due directly to either an excess or a deficiency in one or other of these hormones or both of them.

## Synthetic Oestrogen and Progesterone

The pharmaceutical industry had a financial bonanza and the medical profession an incidental panacea, when the contraceptive pill came into use on a large scale a few years ago and was hailed as the final answer to the problem of birth control. All the different kinds of pill which we have depend for their effectiveness on their content of the two hormones oestrogen and progesterone. The woman who takes the pill is adding a small daily dose of oestrogen and progesterone, in synthetic form, to her body's own production of these substances. The result is a balance of hormones that ordinarily only occurs after a pregnancy has begun. The effect of the additional oestrogen and progesterone is to prevent conception, as would be the case in a normal pregnancy. Nature has so organized the matter that a woman cannot have several foetuses in her womb in various stages of development at the same time.

Physicians soon became aware of the fact that in the contraceptive pill they have a very easy way in which to administer these hormones in the treatment of a number of gynaecological disorders, and in particular, menstrual failure and dysmenorrhoea. Unhappily, there are some doctors who thoughtlessly prescribe the pill for these disorders to young girls, even those in their early teens, as well as to mature women, regardless of what the ultimate consequences might be of employing this hit and miss form of therapy. My regular readers will be aware that I am a vigorous opponent of the pill, whether it be as a contraceptive device or for the treatment of gynaecological disorders, and I am glad to say there are many conscientious doctors who refrain from prescribing it to young girls who fail to menstruate at the appropriate age or suffer from menstrual failure at some time after the onset of menstruation or from painful menstruation. They recognize that it is little short of a crime to interfere with the delicately adjusted endocrine system in these young patients and either recommend the exercise of patience or prescribe some other remedy, should the case be one of dysmenorrhoea.

## Harmful Side Effects

So far as the employment of the pill in the purpose for which it was invented is concerned, from what I learn from association with my patients I am well aware of the many and varied harmful side effects which are so often associated with it. Not surprisingly, in view of its financial implications, the pharmaceutical industry is constantly on the defensive in an attempt to rebut the well-authenticated evidence that this drug can be seriously detrimental to the health of many of the women for whom it is prescribed.

Whilst we condemn the pill, we nevertheless learn a lot from its employment by the medical profession in the treatment of such common ailments as menstrual failure, painful menstruation and pre-menstrual tension. There can be no denying that in these cases it is often very effective. It will often bring on menstruation in cases where young girls have ceased to menstruate as a result of dietary indiscretions and give appreciable relief in some cases of dysmenorrhoea. The trouble is that as soon as the pill is withdrawn the disorder for which it was prescribed will return. Conscientious doctors fully recognize that there is likely to be a grave risk to the long term welfare of the patient in the pill being taken for a lengthy period and will refuse to lend themselves to such a procedure.

There is evidence that it permanently reduces fertility, even after it ceases to be taken, and from time to time it is whispered that it could be cancer-inducing. In this latter connection it is significant that the components of the pill are synthetic in origin and thus are substances which are foreign to the chemical make-up of the body.

Apart from the pill there are, of course, available to the medical profession a number of preparations of oestrogen and progesterone. These are variously employed in the treatment of the unpleasant symptoms arising during a natural or artificial menopause, for inhibiting lactation, or for senile vaginal atrophy.

Progesterone is administered to nullify the effects of excessive oestrogen in habitual abortion. Stilboestrol, considered by some physicians to be the most potent of the oestrogen preparations, has the disadvantage of producing nausea, vomiting and other unpleasant side effects. Many were shocked on being told not long ago in a television programme that this particular hormone, after years of usage, has now been shown to be cancer-inducing.

As a result of extravagant publicity originating in the U.S.A. there is at the present time a big demand among menopausal women for a preparation made from oestrogen derived from the urine of pregnant mares. The claims made for this preparation by its advocates are little short of grotesque. 'No woman need suffer the "change" with its attendant ills and discomfort.' 'No matter what her age may be, no woman need ever feel a day over forty.' When administered under close supervision with the dosage carefully regulated, this remedy does indeed allay menopausal disorders in many cases but most panel doctors refuse to prescribe it. Women with an urge to give this preparation a trial usually have to obtain it as a private patient.

Professor Christopher Dewhurst, Gynaecological Consultant at Queen Charlotte's Hospital has noted that a great deal is claimed for this long-term oestrogen treatment and does not doubt its benefits, but is of the opinion that these are largely emotional. Says the Professor, 'you are not going to keep women young forever by giving oestrogen but they do respond to the feeling of being still hormonally active, not being finished and done with.' He does not discount the cancer risk.

### Hormone Replacement Therapy

From what I have said so far, I think it will be clear that the gynaecological well-being of women and girls depends very much upon their production at the right time of the two hormones oestrogen and progesterone. This must be exactly as nature intended it to be, neither too much nor too little, and in the right proportion. Hormone replacement therapy, as employed by the medical profession, is admitted by doctors themselves to be a very tricky business. So unpredictable are the effects that close supervision is essential if the patient's condition is to be improved rather than worsened. Few panel doctors have time for close supervision of this or any other form of therapy. The long-term effect of administering hormones, whether it be in the form of the contraceptive pill or otherwise, is not known nor will it be known for many years.

Having, I hope, made it clear that hormone replacement therapy, as employed by physicians in the treatment of gynaecological disorders, is open to criticism on a number of counts and, in particular, the potential long-term damage it may cause to the well-being of the patient, it remains to make good my destructive criticism by offering a safer and more acceptable form of therapy which experience has shown to be remarkably effective in many cases.

The remedies at our disposal include herbal medicines and vitamins derived from natural sources. None of them contains hormones but they have the capacity of encouraging the body to produce the hormones in which it is deficient in the right proportion from its own resources.

The first of these remedies is a herbal medicine extracted from a plant native to Mediterranean countries, known as *Vitex Agnus Castus*. A research carried out in the University of Gottingen in Sweden showed that although the Agnus Castus extract does not contain any of the luteal hormone progesterone, nevertheless, through its influence upon the pituitary gland it has the effect of regulating and correcting the balance of this particular hormone in the subject to whom it is administered. As explained later in the chapter, owing to its influence on the pituitary gland, this medicine appears to encourage a correction of hormone deficiency, whether it be of oestrogen or progesterone.

In the case of other herbal remedies by means of which we can seek to correct hormone imbalance, unfortunately, we do not at present have authenticated research to back our belief and our results. All that can be said is that we are in a position to claim, as a result of our experience, that there are herbs which contain precursors of oestrogen, with the result that upon being administered they enable the patient to produce the oestrogen in which she is deficient from her own resources. These oestrogen precursors work in much the same way that pro-vitamin A (Carotene), present in the carrot and some other vegetables, does when it enables the body to produce true vitamin A within the intestines. Some of the herbal extracts we know to be effective when administered in cases of deficiency in this hormone, are: *Aletris farinosa, Chamaelirium luteum, Dioscorea Villosa, Senecio aureus* and *Glycyrrhiza glabra*.

The last mentioned, more familiar as liquorice, although it has the additional virtue of being pleasant to the taste of most people and therefore useful in disguising the somewhat unpleasant taste of some other herbal extracts, has been found in a few cases to encourage weight increase in the same way that the contraceptive pill often does. For this reason it is not given to patients anxious to keep their weight under control. In the case of those desirous of gaining weight there would be an additional benefit.

## Vitamin E

Among the vitamins we have, first and foremost, the controversial vitamin E, subject of the overworked joke among doctors that it promotes fertility in rats. Although it is outside my province here to marshal the overwhelming proof we have of the value of vitamin E in the treatment of a variety of cardiovascular disorders, we have it on the authority of both the Shute brothers, (and Evan Shute is a distinguished gynaecologist,) that vitamin E is an antagonist of oestrogen. Nothing further need be said about this vitamin at the moment, except that if we are to expect good results from its administration the d'alpha tocopherol part of the complex must predominate, it must be derived from natural sources and the dosage must be generous. The last mentioned condition would have to be qualified in cases of high blood-pressure, rheumatic heart disease and diabetes, when it would require to be administered with caution.

Next among the remedies we have that are helpful in the control of hormone balance is seaweed, on account of its appreciable content of natural iodine. Iodine stimulates the thyroid gland to produce its hormones, the chief of which is *thyroxine*. The thyroid hormones are also antagonists of oestrogen.

To return to vitamins, we have it on the authority of the distinguished American endocrinologist, Dr Morton E. Biskind, that vitamin B-complex is also an antagonist of oestrogen. Biskind emphasizes that to be fully effective the whole B-complex must be employed. As a source he favours dessicated liver, because it is unfractionated and thus provides probably the best available source of the, as yet unidentified, factors essential to nutrition. In the case of vegetarians to whom a liver extract would be unacceptable, tablets of B-complex derived from brewer's yeast are readily available. In both cases it is now customary to add $B_{12}$ which is scarce in both liver extract and brewer's yeast. The added $B_{12}$ is a byproduct obtained during the manufacture of antibiotics. I think it certain that the virtue of B-complex is enhanced when we have all its parts.

When, as a practitioner of medical herbalism, I have to consider in what circumstances I should administer the remedies I have described, I think we can assume in the first place that prior to the menopause women are more prone to suffer from over-production of oestrogen, whilst after the menopause their distress is likely to be due to oestrogen deficiency.

The symptoms associated with excess of oestrogen include menorrhagia, dysmenorrhoea with clotting, tension with sore and swollen breasts, weight gain due to fluid retention and liability to develop neoplasms of the breast and uterus. On examination the patient is likely to have a dry skin and hair and a tendency to develop the male type of hair distribution. Our diagnosis of oestrogen excess can usually be verified when we take a cervical and vaginal smear. When examined in the laboratory the cells will tend to be cornified and there will be acidophilic staining in this case. Oestrogen activity would be most marked at the time of ovulation, so the smear should be taken then.

Having satisfied myself that my patient's disorders are due to an excess of oestrogen, I can proceed to administer the oestrogen antagonists at my disposal, namely vitamin E and B-complex, both in generous dosage of not less than 600 i.u. daily in the case of the first and six standardized tablets of the second. A seaweed preparation would also be beneficial, prescribed either in tablets or as a fluid extract.

Since progesterone may also be regarded as an antagonist of oestrogen, further benefit could undoubtedly be expected from prescribing the Agnus Castus preparation, since this medicine has the capacity to encourage progesterone production. In the event of my patient having high blood-pressure or being diabetic, caution would have to be exercised in determining the dosage of vitamin E. One would commence with a small dosage of, say, 200 i.u. daily and progress gradually to the full dosage of 600 i.u. daily over a period of a month or so. In the case of diabetics, the introduction of vitamin E would be likely to call for a reduction in the dosage of insulin, the patient would, therefore, seek the co-operation of the doctor who prescribed this.

It should be mentioned in this connection that those of the medical fraternity who support the employment of vitamin E therapy are highly critical of their colleagues who do not do so where sufferers from diabetes are concerned. They claim that vascular degeneration of the retina of the eye and ultimate blindness, and the tragedy of amputation of legs that have become gangrenous in the elderly could both be avoided by the employment of vitamin E for the prevention of vascular degeneration which so often occurs in elderly cases of diabetes.

## Menopausal Disorders

As I am, unhappily, only too well aware, many women suffer severely from menopausal and post-menopausal disorders, the most common of which are circulatory, bringing about 'hot flushing' and excessive perspiration, especially when in bed at night. The basic cause of these and other menopausal disorders with which one is familiar is undoubtedly oestrogen deficiency. In such cases the anti-oestrogen vitamins which might have been prescribed before the onset of the menopause would be reduced to maintenance level only but the Agnus Castus medication would be continued. Experience has shown that this remedy is very effective in allaying menopausal disorders. The explanation appears to be that as a result of its influence on the pituitary gland, this herb encourages the body to produce the hormones in which it is deficient, whether it be progesterone in the pre-menopause disorders I have described or oestrogen in post-menopausal conditions. I think it would be correct to regard Agnus Castus as a hormone regulator helping to control both an excess or a deficiency of oestrogen, on the one hand, and progesterone on the other.

Together with Agnus Castus we must, when dealing with menopausal disorders, also resort to those medicines which we know to be precursors of oestrogen and which I have already described in detail. These will not have the dramatic results associated with the administration of such a drug as Premarin but in women prepared to exercise patience steady improvement in the condition can be expected and there will be no risk of adverse side effects.

It remains to say something about dysmenorrhoea, menstrual failure and infertility, all of which disorders are, of course, likely to be related either directly or indirectly to the hormone balance of the subject. Painful menstruation, however, can have various direct causes such as under-development or mal-position of the uterus, allergic reaction or psychogenesis. In confining myself to the hormonal implication, it can be said that the disorder could be due to imbalance of either of the hormones with which we are chiefly concerned, oestrogen and progesterone. Under-development of the uterus or the occurrence of clotting would suggest oestrogen deficiency and medication would be organized accordingly. On the other hand, a relative excess of oestrogen and lack of progesterone would be likely to sensitize the uterus to muscular over-activity. When it has been decided, as a result of an investigation, which condition has to be treated, the medication would have to continue for three or four months at least and, thereafter be gradually reduced and finally withdrawn.

I am in no doubt that pre-menstrual tension is due in most cases to progesterone deficiency. It almost always responds favourably to Agnus Castus medication.

As with dysmenorrhoea, so with amenorrhoea or menstrual failure. It can be due to a variety of causes other than endocrine, including pregnancy. The most common cause among patients who come to me for treatment is malnutrition. They are young girls who have sought to control their unwelcome fatty tissue by unwise dieting. Sometimes *anorexia nervosa* also develops and then the outlook can be very serious.

Whether the disorder has been brought about in this way or not, the nutrition of the patient must be raised to a high level by the administration of a balanced course of natural vitamins. Should failure to assimilate nutrients in the diet be suspected, stimulation of the thyroid by giving seaweed extract would be advisable.

### Oestrogen-Progesterone Therapy

In the employment of oestrogen-progesterone therapy there has to be some experimentation over a period of weeks or even months. In the medical profession it is customary, as I have already said, to prescribe both hormones, often for convenience sake, in the form of the contraceptive pill. The more precise physician is likely to administer an oestrogen preparation daily for twenty-one days followed by progesterone for a further five to seven days and, in most cases this will bring on menstruation. This form of treatment has the objection that it has to be continued for several months, during which time the natural processes will have been superseded and weakened, perhaps permanently. In such cases both Agnus Castus and the herbal precursors of oestrogen would be employed by the medical herbalist and the resources of the body would be increased by the prescription of a properly balanced course of natural vitamins. One would also prescribe one or more of the sixteen herbals remedies which are known to encourage menstruation. The treatment of menstrual failure is more fully dealt with in Chapter Six.

Like the preceding disorders dysmenorrhoea and amenorrhoea, infertility suggests much more than a disturbance of the endocrine processes and to do it justice has been made the subject of a separate chapter. (Chapter Eleven).

The time has come to summarize. I consider it logical to prescribe medicines which we believe have the capacity to encourage the body to produce the hormones of which it stands in need in the right proportion and at the right time from its own resources. This form of therapy has a far better chance of being of lasting benefit than that of administering replacement hormones, whether natural or synthetic, as favoured by physicians. These can only have a transient influence for good and could have serious adverse side effects. This is the essence of the matter.

At the same time, we must see to it that as a result of a sensible dietary regime, supplemented by nutrients in concentrated form and derived from natural sources, our patient has available all the elements which may be required to make possible the production of the hormones required on being given the right stimulus.

To avoid disappointment it must be made clear that the herbal medicines to which I have referred would not be available in a health food shop or at a chemist. To obtain treatment by this means you would have to contact a practitioner of herbal medicine, who would be authorized by the Medicines Act to prescribe as necessary. At your health food shop you would be able to obtain all the food and supplements necessary to build up your general health to the high level that would go far to ensure that the medication would be fully effective.

## 14

# VARICOSE VEINS

For reasons not clear to us, women are more liable to develop varicose veins than men, much to their dismay. The disorder is one which women may find hard to bear, not only because varicose veins can be very painful, but perhaps even more so because they are disfiguring. Many a woman's summer holiday has been spoiled by the fact that the unsightliness of the veins in her lower extremities have deterred her from donning a swim suit and joining her husband and children in the pleasures which the seaside offers.

There are grounds for the belief that there is an inherent liability to develop varicose veins. Young girls discuss these matters among themselves and if it so happens that their mothers are afflicted with the disorder they may become very apprehensive that they, themselves, will become victims. Young women in this situation are liable to get into a panic, fearing the worst, when an ominous blue discoloration, and perhaps a slight bulge, appears in the calf of one or both legs, but more about this anon.

When, in the course of his evolution man assumed the upright position, his new vertical posture subjected his venous system, at best relatively vulnerable, to many new burdens.

Our network of veins serves to drain the capillary beds and body tissues of 'used' blood and return this blood to the heart by the rhythmic sucking action of breathing, muscular contraction in the extremities, and valves located in the veins of the legs. If the walls of the veins were rigid, the rhythmic respiratory movements of the chest wall might be sufficient to draw towards it all available blood in the system. As it happens these walls are not rigid, nor are they even similar to the walls of the arteries, which are strongly muscular and elastic.

## One-Way Valves

Gravity assists venous blood from the head and neck to return to the heart. Venous flow from the legs, however, is against the force of gravity, an 'uphill' proposition, and valves which are present in both the deep and superficial veins give an indispensable 'lift' to the returning blood. The valves in our veins are arranged in such a way that blood flows past them towards the heart. They prevent back flow, and are located at regular intervals along the important veins, but generally occur at sites of communication, or junctions, between the deep and the superficial vein systems of the lower extremities. The two sets of veins (deep and superficial) in the leg lie, as their descriptions imply, deeply beneath the skin surface or near to it, respectively.

The superficial set of veins, the *saphenous system*, lies between the deep layers of the leg muscles and the skin, surrounded by subcutaneous fat. The deep set, termed the *femoral veins*, lies between the muscular compartments deep within the leg. These two systems connect in the region of the knee and in the groin. Important valves are present at these junctions. The two systems also connect by a number of communicating veins with valves. In this way the flow of blood can traverse many alternate routes.

## Breakdown of Valves

Varicose veins sufficiently developed to become obvious are obvious indeed, as swollen, tortuous, unsightly bluish cords. Such veins are permanently dilated and there is associated breakdown of the valves within the veins. There will be pain, more or less severe, caused by pressure on adjoining nerves.

The defect responsible for severe varicosities in the legs is failure of the valves to function in communicating veins between the deep and superficial venous systems. When the valves no longer prevent back flow of the column of venous blood, abnormal pressures dilate the superficial venous system, causing stagnation and pooling of the blood.

Statistical comparisons between people whose occupations require much standing and those in sedentary professions reveals no significant difference in the liability to develop varicosities. Prolonged standing may, however, aggravate a pre-existing weakness or proneness towards the formation of varicose veins. Prolonged compression, or constriction of the leg will also contribute to the disorders. Although garters for women have gone out, stockings with elastic tops which followed them were just as bad. Suspender belts and tights do not have the same objection. Women who are allergic to nylon should wear knickers of a different fabric inside their tights.

Varicose veins are liable to appear during pregnancy and may even do so in the early stages before there has been time for pressure to build up in the pelvic region, sufficient to obstruct the venous return. This gives rise to speculation that some other factor may be responsible for the disorder when it happens during pregnancy. In any case, it behoves us to take all the precautions we can to maintain the health of the veins when we have a pregnant woman in our care.

A great disparity often exists between the way varicose veins look and the symptoms they produce. Seldom is there any correlation between the extent of the varicosity that is apparent upon inspection of the leg and the symptoms produced. Not infrequently a leg with insignificant varicosities may cause severe or even excruciating pains, while on the other hand, some legs with numerous and unsightly varicose veins may not cause appreciable discomfort.

## Early Symptoms

As a general rule, varicose veins may cause symptoms of tenseness and burning, or itching of the skin. Other early symptoms are heaviness, a drawing sensation and a cramping feeling in the calf of the leg. Often after long standing the legs feel heavy or have a sensation of numbness. Severe and prolonged pain is not likely to occur unless there is ulceration or phlebitis.

When it comes to treatment the orthodox medical profession — in cases which are not severe — will recommend the use of some form of elastic stocking for support and perhaps the injection into the veins of a chemical which will have the effect of putting them out of action. The principle of the elastic stocking is simple. Elastic pressure upon the dilated veins forces blood into other venous channels which can more effectively carry it towards the heart. The injection treatment has a similar result. It must be pointed out that both methods of treatment are palliatives only, and do not in any way get to the root of the trouble. There is the further objection, especially to injections, that the skin and the tissue beneath it is deprived of nutrition and thus there is a very real risk of complications developing. The local malnutrition may well cause inflammation or even thrombophlebitis. The skin appearance will vary from a brownish leathery discoloration to an acutely inflamed reddish burning aspect. Thus varicose dermatitis is a frequent forerunner of ulceration.

The operation of choice advocated by the medical profession for the treatment of varicose veins consists of the tying off and removal of the main *saphenous* vein and others involved. It includes individual tying and division of any incompetent communicating or perforating veins that might tend to compromise the results of operation. In addition, the great saphenous vein is stripped and in this way the entire dilated or tortuous vein is removed.

The Canadian Medical Protective Association annually warns doctors to consider the operation of ligation and stripping of veins as 'one of the most potentially dangerous any patient may have to undergo because of the irreversible results which generally follow error . . . It is only part of the answer to say that vein stripping should be done only by skilled, experienced surgeons . . . it can be demonstrated that skill is not enough, as witness the fact that some of these difficulties have arisen at the hands of the most highly skilled and widely respected practitioners.' Recurrence rates are high after surgical treatment.

We, the unorthodox, are constantly complaining that the medical profession are far more concerned with treating the symptoms of a disorder than in eliminating its cause. The stripping of varicose veins is a classic example of this tendency. If nature, in her wisdom, deemed it necessary to provide the lower limbs with these important veins for their welfare it is hard to see how their removal can be beneficial in the long run. It is obvious that the areas nearest the surface will be deprived of adequate drainage and suffer damage in consequence. In point of fact nature will make an effort to replace the missing veins but it has frequently been shown that these too will become varicosed sooner or later if nothing is done to remove the cause of the congestion.

**Injudicious Diet**

The development of varicose veins, and also related disorders, such as varicocele and haemorrhoids, has been shown very convincingly by a medical doctor, oddly enough, and not as we might expect by a naturopath, to be due in the main to an injudicious diet. Surgeon-Captain T.L. Cleave has explained his theory in a number of books and it is a very simple one. The custom so common today of removing much of the fibre from cereals, and the whole of it from sugar cane and sugar beet, frequently leads to an unnatural delay in the passage of the contents of the colon and hence to an increase in the size (through expansion) and weight. Since a relatively small pressure can arrest the blood flow in even the largest veins, the intimate relationship of the colon to the veins that run past it on the way to the heart, can easily produce an obstructive effect in them and hence ultimately to varicose veins through back pressure.

The fact that many people suffering from varicose veins would not admit to any difficulty with the bowel counts for little. Many people consider that the bowel is acting normally if they pass a stool each day, whereas the true criteria of normality are the diameter and hardness in the stool passed, which increases steadily with delay. A person who considers the bowel is acting normally just because he or she passes a stool each day may, in fact, always be suffering from a twenty-four hours, or more, delay. Therefore, instead of seeking the cause of varicose veins in simple constipation, it is necessary to seek it in *a delayed rate of passage of the colonic contents, as opposed to the natural rate.* The italics appear in Surgeon-Captain Cleave's own writings.

The remedy is a simple one. It is to remove the cause of the obstruction in the circulation, by changing — through dieting — the character of the stools, both as regards diameter and hardness. The diet must aim at restoring fibre in foods and not in the use of aperients. Restitution can often be achieved by simply and pleasantly switching from white bread and other foods containing white flour to true wholemeal bread and other foods containing true wholemeal flour, and as far as possible from ordinary refined sugar, and the various sweetstuffs containing it; to fruits and vegetables whether fresh or dried (but not tinned). The substitution of wholemeal flour for white flour is both essential and easy, provided the great pitfall is avoided of being served with 'brown' bread or flours which are not really wholemeal at all, having had varying quantities of the bran removed. White sugar in foods should be totally abandoned as far as practicable and an unrefined sugar, such as Barbados, substituted as necessary. Honey may also be used for sweetening. Muesli is very suitable as a breakfast food and bran even more so, because of its value as a roughage.

If a positive desire for health is present it is perfectly feasible to achieve a substantial amount of this substitution, and certainly enough to produce a radical change in the action of the bowels. When making the change in diet to include more roughage the importance of thorough mastication must be borne in mind, otherwise indigestion with flatulence will result.

Besides making a radical change in diet, which is the first step in the right direction, there is much else that can be done to arrest the development of varicose veins and bring about amelioration when they are already troublesome.

We have abundant evidence that a specific remedy in the treatment of varicose veins is vitamin E (d'alpha tocopherol) provided it is genuinely derived from natural sources. The purpose of treatment with vitamin E is not so much to shrink the varicosities, but to alleviate the symptoms from within. The distended and tortuous veins cause a chronic venous stasis which produces a swelling, stabbing and aching pain, and if severe enough and prolonged enough, will result in ulceration, overgrowth of connective tissue and occasionally leakage of blood under the skin. Vitamin E therapy almost always completely removes the aches and pains by decreasing the oxygen need of the tissues involved, whilst by opening up effective collateral circulation, it also reduces the swelling. At the commencement of treatment the dosage of vitamin E would be six capsules of 100 i.u. per day reduced after six months to half this quantity as a maintenance dosage.

Supporting therapy in the form of herbal and homoeopathic remedies would speed the alleviation of the disorder and reduce liability to relapse. Among remedies commonly prescribed are *Majorana* (Marjoram), *Aloes, Hamamelis Virg.* (Witch Hazel), *Sanguisorba off.* (Burnet), *Calendula off.* (Marigold), and *Symphytum off.* (Comfrey).

A helpful measure of self-treatment is vigorous daily dry brushing of the legs. When the pain is severe, relief can be obtained by spraying the area with cold water. The foot of the bed can be raised a few inches on blocks.

In addition to prescribing suitable herbal or homoeopathic remedies, your practitioner would almost certainly give you a special form of manipulative treatment with a view to improving the circulation and would also teach you some simple exercises. In the event of a displacement of the uterus being a contributary cause, steps would have to be taken to put this right.

Finally, when girls and young women become aware of the

ominous signs mentioned in the early part of this chapter, it would be wise to seek early advice and if necessary, early treatment before marked unsightliness has had time to develop.

## 15

## CERVICITIS, POLYPS AND PRURITUS

The disorders which I shall discuss in this chapter are, unfortunately, all too common in women. Symptoms such as *leucorrhoea* (abnormal vaginal discharge) and *pruritus* (severe genital itching) would seem to give rise to worry and distress more frequently than any other, if the letters I receive are anything to go by.

The cervix is that part of the womb which projects into the vagina and is in shape rather like the small end of a pear with the stalk pulled out to simulate the entrance. Although small in area, it is one of the most important organs from the point of view of gynaecological health and the avoidance of malignancy. All women nowadays are well aware of the vulnerability of the cervix because they are constantly being urged to have a cervical smear taken in order to determine whether or not the cervix is free from traces of potential malignancy. To be forewarned is to be forearmed, therefore such lesions of the cervix as cervicitis, erosions, polyps, cysts and lacerations should be regarded as warning signals and treatment sought without delay.

If you have a polyp it may have been there for months or even years and you could be totally unaware of it until it is discovered in the course of a gynaecological examination, but sometimes polyps give rise to intermittent bleeding and to a vaginal discharge which we call leucorrhoea. They vary in size from that of a pin's-head to a length of an inch or more. I once had a patient with a polyp on the vulva, a very unusual position, which was larger than a walnut. In appearance the more common polyps are like little pear-shaped bags attached by a stalk. They are smooth and soft and reddish or purplish in colour. It is unusual for there to be more than one polyp. They often have a large number of small blood vessels. If these are near the surface, intermittent bleeding may occur but in some cases polyps have a tough exterior and do not give rise to bleeding or any other symptoms, and are virtually harmless. Polyps are liable to become inflamed in cases where the vaginal secretions are unhealthy.

The structure of the cervix is unusually complicated, with

clefts and folds owing, no doubt, to its liability to be called upon to perform a prodigious stretching act in the event of childbirth.

## Bacterial Infection

The intricate structure of the organ requires cell renewal at a greater rate than in other parts of the body. When it is desired to obtain discarded cells for laboratory examination, whilst taking a cervical smear, there will always be plenty available. It is probably due to its intricate structure that the cervix is particularly susceptible to bacterial infection by such organisms as *gonococcus, streptococcus, staphylococcus* and *escherichia coli.* One or other of these infections usually follow some kind of trauma, such as that of childbirth, instrumental dilation, curettage, improper treatment by cauterization and so on, but it is important to bear in mind that these infections would not make much headway if the vaginal secretions were truly healthy.

An erosion may be present all round the cervical entrance or only part way round. Usually with this condition there is an excessive amount of mucus secretion and in some cases the mucosal folds become obstructed and cause cysts to form. They, in turn, may interfere with the circulation and give rise to the bleeding which occurs sometimes just before and just after menstruation, and also an unpleasant vaginal discharge at other times. In many cases of cervicitis (as we call the condition), there is an associated inflammation within the womb and in the ligaments that support the organ, when the latter structures will feel tender to touch in the lower abdomen.

The most obvious symptom of cervicitis is the discharge, technically known as leucorrhoea, which is present in almost every case. Other symptoms may be a 'bearing down' feeling in the pelvis, backache, dull pain in the lower part of the abdomen and urinary disturbances, especially over-frequency and urgency of urination. In some cases there may also be menstrual irregularity. Women with cervicitis usually complain of painful intercourse. A rather frequent consequence of the disorder is sterility and this is not surprising, for sperm can hardly be expected to behave normally in such an unfavourable environment. It has been noted that many women who have been slow to conceive do so after the cervicitis has been cured.

If you go to a doctor and he decides, after investigation, that you have a cervical polyp, he will refer you to a hospital and the treatment you will receive there at the hands of the gynaecologists will be surgical removal of the growth. If there is bleeding this will probably be dealt with by applying an electric cautery tip to the site. I have yet to hear of any attempt being made to advise the patient how the formation of further polyps might be prevented.

In the case of erosions and other forms of cervicitis, some consideration is given to prevention by orthodox gynaecologists. It is pointed out that in a considerable proportion of cases the disorder is a result of a venereal disease, usually gonorrhoea, therefore, measures to reduce the incidence of gonorrhoea are advocated. Also advocated is more patience in delivering women of their babies. When spontaneous deliveries without the use of drugs or instruments are encouraged, there may not occur the severe lacerations of the cervix and the perineum of which so many mothers are victims. Not only do they suffer pain and discomfort from adhesions for months, or even years, after delivery, but the fissures which result provide an ideal breeding ground for the pathological organisms with which we are concerned.

### Cauterization: After-Effects
Some of the more thoughtful and patient gynaecologists will go so far as to agree that therapeutic lotions are worth trying and may yield good results, but the majority will lose no time in resorting to cauterization. The instrument most often used is an electric cautery. The cervix is exposed to view by the insertion of an instrument called a speculum. The tip of the cautery is placed on the affected area and the current is turned on. After the tip becomes red hot the inflamed area is burnt away. Sometimes, but not always, the patient is told what after-effects of cauterization she may expect. These could be a profuse discharge which may go on for days or even weeks, and may be tinged with blood. Sometimes there is much bleeding, which will require separate treatment. Backache often follows treatment by cauterization and may persist for a long time. Please note that these details of the possible after-effects of cauterization are not figments of my imagination, calculated to frighten my readers. I am quoting from a standard work on gynaecology.

When we have to treat polyps or cervicitis in accordance with naturopathic principles, the first consideration is to restore the health of the vaginal secretions. It is not seriously disputed by physiologists that these, and many other gynaecological disorders, are triggered off and aggravated as a result of hormone imbalance. Almost all major events in life happen under the influence of hormones. Their action is unpredictable when used as a drug. For that reason it will be readily apparent that we would probably be fighting a losing battle if, at the commencement of treatment, we did not ban the use of the contraceptive pill by our patient. The first principle of naturopathic treatment is to remove the causes of the ailment and, without doubt, this is one of them.

It is now fully recognized that the most common cause of *pruritus valvae* in women is the existence of a micro-organism known as *Trichomonas Vaginalis*. Infestation causes redness, usually associated with burning, irritation and chafing of the skin in the region of the vulva. Sometimes there is severe itching.

### Therapeutic Jelly

Trichomonas cannot thrive if the natural secretions of the vagina are healthy and the acid/alkaline balance normal. This being so, the most promising treatment is to restore the health of the secretions by use of a therapeutic jelly which the patient can quite easily introduce herself, if she is provided with the means. At the same time, herbal or homoeopathic medicine can be prescribed in order to accelerate the progress of the treatment and reduce the likelihood of a recurrence at some later date.

The remedies the practitioner would be likely to favour would be those related to inflammation of the vagina and vulva (vulvovaginitis) in general. They include *Chenopodium Olidum, Thuja Occidentalis, Santalam Album* and *Copaiba.*

It is unlikely that these herbs would be available in your health food shop and certainly not at a chemist. Since the blending and the question whether to administer in medicinal or homoeopathic dosage and potency must be considered in each case, self-treatment would not be a practicable proposition.

The therapeutic jelly for vaginal injection would also need to be prescribed and supplied by a practitioner.

The next most common cause of vulvovaginitis, giving rise to pruritus, is what we call a 'yeast infection'. Sometimes this is referred to as 'thrush' but the medical designation is *Candida*

*Albicans.* In this case the discharge is more often found in pregnant women and in the elderly and in association with diabetes and there may be little or no itching. The malady arises from a fungus invasion for which we have another name: *Moniliasis.*

For the effective treatment of this disorder the same herbal prescriptions as in the case of Trichomonas are indicated, but a different kind of medicinal jelly for vaginal introduction would be required, and used night and morning for a period of at least fourteen days.

The components of this and the previously mentioned therapeutic jelly, although not herbal, have been in regular use for a very long time and are quite harmless and without side-effects. They are, in fact, very soothing. The incidence of allergic manifestations which could be attributed to this form of therapy is extremely rare.

Many women are much distressed after the change of life has occurred, when they find the vagina entrance becoming extremely sensitive and irritable and liable to intermittent bouts of pruritus. This state of affairs is basically due to changes in the hormone balance associated with the menopause, and this, in turn, brings about a wasting or atrophy of tissue of the vagina and loss of elasticity, especially near the entrance.

As with infections of the vagina such as Trichomonas and Candida, the employment of a therapeutic jelly can again be resorted to with profit, whilst some soothing herbal ointment will be additionally helpful. Fortunately, there is available a herbal medicine which has the capacity to correct the hormone balance through its influence on the pituitary (or master) gland. Of course, it is not itself a hormone.

### Hormones Rashly Prescribed

We medical herbalists are extremely critical of the all-too-ready prescription by medical doctors of synthetic hormones, both for therapeutic purposes and in the form of the contraceptive pill. This is because women vary so much in their reactions to hormones. The end result is quite unpredictable. It comes about with disturbing frequency that the side-effects resulting from taking hormones are a great deal harder to bear and damaging to health, than the ailment they are supposed to cure. They are particularly harmful when administered to young girls, in whom the gynaecological balance can be so easily upset. To give you an idea how rashly hormones are used nowadays by some physicians, usually for convenience sake in the form of the contraceptive pill, I will recount a recent incident. A woman phoned to say she was extremely worried about her daughter, aged thirteen-and-a-half years, who was in the process of having her first menstruation. It turned out to be very heavy with clotting and after ten days had not stopped. The girl had been taken to the local G.P. when, to her mother's horror, he prescribed 'the pill'.

She refused to let her daughter take this remedy and it was at this stage when she phoned me. The girl was brought to see me, when a brief examination revealed no organic disorder. I am pleased to say she responded satisfactorily to herbal therapy and had no further menstrual trouble.

Pruritus of the anal passage is much less common than *pruritus vaginalis* and, for some reason or other, appears to occur more often in men than in women. When men are infected it could be that the disorder has been transmitted from their partner in sexual relations. It should be remarked, in this connection, that when one is treating a case of *pruritus vaginalis* in a woman, which proves to be very resistant to the regular forms of therapy, the fact must not be lost sight of that whilst a man can be infected by a woman the reverse can also be the case, although the offending organism was almost certainly nurtured originally in the vaginal secretions of the woman.

Attention to hygiene in the male should be sufficient to protect him from infection by his marital partner and to make it unlikely that he will harbour the offending organism.

*Pruritus ani* can also be due to worms, haemorrhoids, diabetes or anal fissures, and when it occurs one must, as in any other ailment, seek the cause and prescribe such treatment as may be necessary.

## 16

## AILMENTS OF THE URINARY SYSTEM

Cystitis! A most unpleasant ailment much dreaded by women, in whom it is all-too-common. In writing something about it and other disorders of the urinary system we must begin with the two kidneys. These are glandular organs situated close to the spine in the upper part of the abdominal cavity. The main function of the kidneys is to separate fluids and some solids from the blood. It is estimated that each day no less than 500 pints of blood can be dealt with by these small organs, only weighing about 4 oz each.

The bulk of the filtrate — after passing through the kidneys — is returned to the blood stream, but unwanted products, which the body wishes to reject, dissolved in water, are excreted in the form of urine by the way of two tubes which we call ureters. The ureters empty their contents into the bladder, where it is stored until such time as it is found convenient to finally excrete it by urination. The average amount of urine excreted each day by an adult is three pints.

In the process of urination a valve-like muscle called the sphincter is opened at the base of the bladder at the will of the subject. Urine passes out by way of another tube called the urethra. In a woman this tube is only about 1½ inches long. It emerges in the vulva about half-an-inch below the clitoris and between it and the vaginal entrance.

### Frequent Micturition: Causes
Since we are not directly concerned in this chapter with diseases of the kidneys themselves, we will begin our consideration of ailments with morbid states of the bladder causing frequent and painful micturition.

Frequent desire to pass water, with a varying amount of incontinence or involuntary leakage, is often the result of prolapse of the vaginal walls, which causes the urethra to be pushed out of its normal position. Full control is then lost and urine escapes involuntarily after coughing, sneezing or running.

Another common cause of frequency of micturition is cystocele. This is a hernia or prolapse of the bladder, which then sags into the vagina. A bladder pouch is thus formed in which urine remains, causing irritation and a frequent desire to pass water.

In very severe cases of urethra displacement, cystocele and bladder prolapse, surgery is the only remedy likely to give substantial relief, provided the operation is skilfully carried out. Less serious cases will respond well to less drastic forms of treatment which you can obtain from a naturopath or medical herbalist. When such a practitioner has examined you he will be able to advise you what is necessary and will not refer you to a surgeon unless this is clearly the only reasonable solution.

It is important to bear in mind in this connection that surgery does not necessarily remove the cause of the disorder. There may be an aftermath of complications if your surgeon is not a skilful one. A naturopath will seek to improve the situation by teaching you exercises to strengthen the musculature, by manipulative treatment designed to enhance local circulation and, if he is also a medical herbalist, by prescribing suitable remedies that will work from within.

Sufferers from these disorders should at all times make an effort to empty the bladder completely at each micturition. After passing urine they should wait a minute or two and then try again to make sure the bladder is really empty. By encouraging the bladder to expel its contents more completely, the impetus to urinate is removed for a longer period.

Many women complain of frequent desire to urinate disturbing their sleep, for even in the absence of physical defects there are still those who have to get up once or more every night. Some further explanation must be sought in cases of this kind. It will usually be found on investigation that either the bladder has acquired 'bad habits' or that the intake of fluid at or near bedtime is excessive.

Most important is the influence of habit in the case of the patient who awakens at the same hour each night with an urgent desire to urinate. The effect of position must not be overlooked. Lying on the back may be the means of evoking a functional reaction culminating in a desire to pass water, the desire disappearing when the patient turns on her side. The effect of lying on the back may often be observed in children who have not yet realized that relief may be obtained by the simple expedient of turning on the side.

In adults relief must not only be sought by alteration of the sleeping position, but still more by striving to break the habit through making a genuine effort to retain the urine in the bladder until getting-up time. Urine should be passed before beginning to undress and a further attempt be made before getting into bed.

The fluid we drink takes longer to find its way via the kidneys into the bladder than we realize. Some sufferers with the problem we are discussing have found by experiment that it is not so much the fluid that is drunk at bedtime that causes the trouble as the afternoon cups of tea. I suggest a trial be made by those who think it worth while in avoiding all fluid between the mid-day meal and a late supper and see what happens.

## Cystitis

All too often women suffer from inflammation of the bladder, that most distressing disorder which we call cystitis. This can be acute or chronic. The acute version, which often comes on suddenly and with great severity, is usually due to an infection of some kind, or through exposure to cold and dampness. Getting the feet and legs wet or sitting on a cold surface may bring on an attack.

In an acute attack of cystitis there will be severe local pain, scalding during and after urination, small quantities of urine containing pus being passed on each occasion, and in very acute stages, some blood. There is often a rise in temperature and the patient feels and looks ill.

During an attack the patient should rest in bed and subsist on a mainly liquid diet. Barley water, which has a soothing influence, should be drunk freely whilst alcohol should be avoided altogether; also condiments and spices. Hot sitz baths will be found comforting and may be taken several times daily. Chamomile, a herb obtainable at most health food shops, can be added to the bath water with profit. The liquid diet might include fruit and vegetable juices as well as milk.

Chronic or recurrent cystitis may follow an acute attack, especially if the cause of the ailment is not discovered and removed. Causes include an infection called *trichomonas vaginalis* very common in women, *bacillus coli* infection which is less common, diabetes or a kidney disorder. The possibility of venereal disease cannot be excluded.

When there is a bacterial infection such as trichomonas or possibly a fungoid one, of which *candida albicans* is an example, the seat will be within the vagina and it will not then be a bladder infection. The patient will be required to use a therapeutic paste or jelly for some time. This is injected into the vagina by means of an applicator.

Its purpose is to correct the acid/alkaline balance of the vaginal secretions and improve the local environment in general, so that the bacteria responsible for the infection can no longer thrive and will disappear. This treatment will have to be persevered with for three or four weeks or even longer in resistant cases. The disorder can also be attacked from within by prescribing suitable herbal or homoeopathic remedies. (See Chapter Fifteen).

When the infection is really one of the bladder, and probably due to another kind of bacteria, such as *coli*, the treatment will primarily require the administration of herbal or homoeopathic remedies, which we recognize as natural antibiotics. These, whilst being very effective, have no harmful side-effects and can be taken for a long enough period to rid the patient of the bacillis. One of the most effective of these remedies is derived from the seeds of that humble flower, the nasturtium.

When the practitioner has reason to believe there is a kidney disorder he will confirm this by the testing of a urine sample and may then initiate a different kind of treatment.

Women who are prone to contract cystitis should make it a habit always to wear warm under-clothes and never to sit on a cold, damp seat. Young girls wearing mini-skirts will need something more than tights under these in cold weather.

In *urethritis* there is inflammation of the urethra, arising also from an infection. The practitioner in the course of his examination will confirm that this is present if he is able to express pus from the organ by squeezing and otherwise manipulating it. It will be necessary to treat the infection locally, perhaps with a lotion of *Calendula*, as well as giving a remedy to combat the ailment from within.

Frequency of micturition is often associated with pregnancy, especially in its early and late stages.

A more serious condition which sometimes occurs in pregnancy is abnormal retention of urine and this can have serious consequences if not relieved by the administration of suitable treatment. Remedies of choice might be *Terebinthina* or *Aconitum* and the patient would be asked to sit in a shallow hot bath so as to apply heat in the appropriate area at frequent intervals.

### 'Irritable Bladder'

The term 'irritable bladder' is sometimes applied to a condition often existing in single women who have reached or passed middle age. There are frequent calls to pass water during the day as well as during the night. Usually no direct cause can be discovered and thus amelioration or cure can be a matter of considerable difficulty. The simple explanation would appear to be, as was the case when we referred to the habit interfering with a night's rest, that the bladder has contracted bad habits.

As a temporary measure homoeopathic doses of *Nux Vomica* or *Uva Ursi* may be prescribed. It may turn out that the disorder is not merely one of bad habit but of upset, temporary or permanent, of the neuromuscular mechanism of the bladder, in which case the teaching of simple exercises will be the most promising remedy.

In young girls great distress is caused if they have the misfortune to contract *vulvo-vaginitis*, an infection which brings about severe irritation of the vulva and hymen accompanied by a discharge. It seems to be caught through sitting on a lavatory seat which has been infected by adults. Girls should be warned, when they have to use strange lavatories, to cover the front of the seat with toilet paper before sitting down.

In treating *vulvo-vaginitis* nothing should be applied locally excepting *Chickweed* ointment, which is very soothing, or *Calendula* ointment, which has wonderful healing properties. The girl should rest in bed during the acute stage of the attack and should have warm hip baths at least twice daily. After each bath, *Chickweed* or *Calendula* ointment should be applied, the choice depending on which gives the greatest relief.

Should there be more than one attack the girl might be taken to a medical herbalist or naturopath for an examination and professional treatment. The medical herbalist would prescribe remedies designed to attack the infection at its source by way of the blood stream.

Many parents will be familiar with a distressing disorder occurring in both girls and boys, *nocturnal enuresis* or, more familiarly, bed wetting. The habit can be due to many causes, the most common of which in older children is mental strain, induced by over-stimulation of the brain through excessive school work and being driven by parents to make greater efforts in that direction.

Preliminary treatment should include a daily cold sitz bath to tone up the bladder, or if this seems too drastic, the parts in the region of the bladder should receive a daily sponging with cold water. Sympathy and avoidance of undue strictness is important in these cases.

To prevent abnormally deep sleep, the child should be awakened once or twice during the night and caused to pass urine. Fluids in the late afternoon and evening should be reduced to a minimum or stopped altogether. The bed should not be too soft.

In obstinate cases I have found a blended homoeopathic remedy including *Hypericum, Chamomile, Pulsatilla* and *Valarian* very effective.

A final word concerning both sexes, but especially girls. They should be brought up not to be unreasonably shy about going to a lavatory as soon as the need is felt. If the bladder is frequently over-stretched it is liable to have its natural functioning damaged. From this a life-long history of incontinence can result.

In a girl, frequent over-filling of the bladder is also liable to result in an early displacement of the womb, which could be a source of trouble for the rest of her days.

## 17

# TREATING UTERINE FIBROIDS WITHOUT SURGERY

Fibroid tumours are the most common form of tumour likely to develop in various parts of the body. In women they are far more apt to be found within or outside the uterus than elsewhere, with the exception of the breasts. Fibroid tumours consist of masses of muscle fibre, similar to that of the uterus itself, and white fibrous tissue. They vary in size from that of a small pea to a mass weighing several pounds and as large as a full-term pregnancy. Quite often the tumours are multiple and knobbly and cause the womb to be not unlike a lumpy potato, with nodules buried in its wall.

It is estimated that some 20 per cent of women of thirty-five years of age or over have these abnormal growths. They are characteristic of sexual maturity, the majority occurring in the third, fourth or fifth decades. The cause is not known, but they are more common in women who have never borne children than those with children. There is a saying that the womb has an urge to produce. If it does not produce babies, as it was designed to do, it will produce something else. Although a uterine fibroid can first make its appearance at any time between puberty and the menopause it is usually first recognized between the ages of 30 and 45. The symptoms depend upon the size and site of the tumour, and many fibroids give rise to no symptoms at all. Pain is seldom a marked feature.

It quite often happens that a fibroid is first discovered during a physical examination when a woman attends a practitioner for a gynaecological check-up. There may have been disordered menstruation, sterility, frequency of micturition, and a vague discomfort, but she has not considered these symptoms might be attributable to a tumour.

If the fibroid or fibroids are not large and cause little or no pressure or menstrual abnormalities and no pain, treatment should be aimed at arresting development and this is where we find a marked difference in the attitudes of the orthodox and unorthodox gynaecologist. The former will either suggest that the patient should have an operation straight away or ask her to return after six months to find out what development there has been in the meantime. Nothing will be done to arrest development and it is, therefore, almost inevitable — if the patient has not begun the menopause — that the fibroid will increase in size, quite rapidly in some cases, until eventually a surgical operation will be unavoidable. It is rare for uterine fibroids to be malignant.

### The Ovarian Cyst
The ovaries, as well as the uterus, are liable to invasion by growths, the majority of which are benign in character. The most common form of abnormal growth in these organs is the ovarian cyst. This is a sac containing fluid or fibrous matter. Small cysts sometimes disappear, especially if appropriate treatment is given as soon as they are detected. A cyst that has a slender stem (or *pedicle*) may twist tightly around the stem, giving rise to abdominal pain very similar to that caused by appendicitis.

The ovaries, as well as being producers of eggs, also produce sex hormones, one of which is estrogen, and the other is progesterone. Their function is primarily to regulate menstruation and maintain the uterus in a favourable condition for conception and child bearing. In some cases the presence of an ovarian cyst will seriously interfere with the normal control of hormone production and thus give rise to a variety of unpleasant symptoms, including painful and irregular menstruation.

Owing to their possible nearness to each other, it can be difficult for the gynaecologist to determine whether his patient has an ovarian cyst or a uterine fibroid but a comparison of the accompanying symptoms will offer him a fairly reliable clue. Sometimes when surgery is resorted to, and the abdomen of the patient is opened, both an ovarian cyst and a uterine fibroid, or fibroids, will be disclosed.

### Treatment or Surgery?
When consulted by women who are affected with tumours and cysts, the naturopathic gynaecologist is faced with the responsibility of making a decision whether he should undertake treatment with the means at his disposal or recommend that his patient should submit to surgery. The value of gynaecological examinations carried out regularly at yearly, or two-yearly intervals will be appreciated when I point out that much will

depend on the stage of development of the disorder. If a large fibroid or cyst is found and it is clear that this is responsible for a variety of symptoms which give rise to a great deal of distress, and if at the same time the patient is nearing the onset of the menopause, it would be the clear duty of the practitioner to prepare her to face the ordeal of surgical removal. Quite understandably, most women dread the prospect of major surgery involving the opening of the abdomen. When this is inevitable we have to give them all the moral support we can and at the same time use our offices, when circumstances permit, to ensure the operation will be carried out in such a way as to cause the minimum of distress. Although hysterectomies (total removal of the womb) are carried out far too freely in some hospitals, the average woman is never quite the same afterwards, whilst in cases where both ovaries are removed her whole character may be changed to her detriment and to the consternation of her nearest and dearest, because her hormone balance has been most distastrously upset.

A surgeon who is both skilful and conscientious will do his best to save as much as possible of all these organs.

Where orthodox medicine fails lamentably is in preparing the patient for the operation and in restoring her to good health thereafter. This is a matter to which I attach the greatest importance, for the results can be extremely rewarding. By means of judicious dieting aided by the prescription of a balanced course of natural vitamins and, in some cases, a herbal or homoeopathic tonic, vitality can be built up wonderfully well, whilst the performance of some simple exercises will help matters in other ways. I have known many cases of women who have had proper pre-operative and post-operative treatment being quite amazed when they have compared themselves with other surgical patients who have had no such assistance. Almost always there is a marked absence of unpleasant and distressing after-effects in our patients whilst recovery of full health is far more speedy. I often think it is in this sphere that we do some of our most rewarding work.

Let us now consider the patient in whom we have located a fibroid tumour which, in our opinion, does not warrant surgical removal. Clearly it is of the greatest importance that any development of the disorder should be arrested. If regression is also achieved, so much the better.

## Walking, Running and Games

As always in naturopathy, the best form of treatment is removal of the cause. In almost all gynaecological disorders poor circulation and inadequate elimination is at the root of the trouble. The reason an ever-increasing number of women, both young and old, find themselves in hospital suffering from serious gynaecological ailments is undoubtedly the unnatural way they have lived. Like the rest of us they ride about in motor cars and other vehicles a great deal, whilst only a minimum of travelling is done on foot. Walking should be regarded as the most natural form of exercise but we get very little of it. It would seem that fewer girls and young women play games such as tennis and badminton than used to be the case, though maybe more ride horses, which is not quite so beneficial. Walking and running and the playing of games, by reason of the rhythmic movements thereby brought about, serve to accelerate the circulation of the blood to all the organs of the body, including those of reproduction. If movement of the uterus is brought about in this way from childhood upwards, the ligaments which support it will be better developed and in better tone and the uterus itself and the whole environment will be in better case. When called upon to carry out gynaecological examinations I can usually distinguish the sedentary type of woman from the active one. Unfortunately, now that so many women and girls spend hours of their lives travelling in trains, buses and cars to offices where they sit for more hours, the former predominate.

## Sub-Nutrition

On top of this unhealthy state of affairs in the physical sphere we have, all too often, the further disadvantage of what might be called sub-nutrition. From babyhood upwards the majority of women subsist on overprocessed and unnutritious foods loaded with chemical additives in which carbohydrates predominate. Quite apart from lowering the vigour and general well-being of the subject, this regime almost always results in chronic constipation and this is probably the worst of all the enemies of gynaecological health. The predominence of carbohydrates often results in young girls putting on weight and this they are liable to regard as a misfortune of the first magnitude. They embark upon a slimming regime without proper supervision, with the inevitable result that menstruation ceases and then we have a real disaster. We have to treat girls in this predicament all too often and, believe me, it is no easy matter to get menstruation started again when it has stopped as the result of unsupervised and injudicious dieting.

Removal of the causes of gynaecological disorders requires, in the first place, that the circulation of the blood be improved. The blood stream performs the all-important functions of eliminating from the body, and all its organs, the waste products of its activities. Millions of cells reach their life span and are discarded every day. Not only does the circulating blood collect these and carry them away to be eliminated through the urine, the faeces and the pores of the skin, but it provides also the nutriments from which new cells are formed to replace the worn-out ones which have been discarded. All forms of tumour, of ulcer and of skin disease are, in fact, indications of abnormal elimination or failure to eliminate. Because the blood is not doing its work efficiently, nature has to provide a different means of getting rid of toxic matter, otherwise the host would die of toxic poisoning.

In order to improve the circulation a gynaecological patient must receive a properly organized course of treatment. Light osteopathic manipulation must be given in particular to the spine and abdomen. Special exercises are taught, with emphasis on correct breathing and the development and conscious control of the musculature in the reproductive area. The uterus itself must be given a specialized form of manipulation. This is because almost always when the gynaecological health is poor the uterus will be found to be misplaced, lacking mobility and tone and generally unhealthy.

It is not sufficient to restore efficient circulation of the blood and do nothing to improve its quality. The diet of the patient must be fully considered and improved if necessary. Almost always, at a time when it is so difficult to obtain truly wholesome and nutritious foods, there will be a marked deficiency in some of the vital substances. This must be rectified by prescribing minerals and vitamins derived from natural sources, not in a haphazard manner but in proper balance.

The vital forces of the body will decline and may become inactive when efficient elimination and adequate nutrition has been neglected. We medical herbalists have at our disposal a great variety of herbal and homoeopathic medicines which will serve to unlock these vital forces, so that they can play their full part in the restoration of health. These remedies are safe and free from side-effects and thus totally different in their action from the powerful drugs now employed by orthodox medicine — employed, it would seem, to spectacularly suppress the symptoms which are presented without doing anything to remove their cause. Many doctors are in agreement that this is not good therapy.

A correct diet is extremely important in the treatment of fibroids. If the patient is over-weight, immediate steps must be taken to reduce weight, first to what is normal for the height and build of the subject and thereafter to a few pounds below normal. This procedure will inhibit the growth of the tumour by depriving it of nourishment.

**Principle of Autolysis**
Autolysis, or self-destruction of tissue, when applied to the treatment of such disorders as fibroids, depends for its successful working on the well-substantiated principle that the body, when cell-building nutrients (protein) at its disposal are below the optimum level, will always maintain its vital tissues from what is available before it will nourish pathological tissue. We must, of course, include tumours in this category. It is my experience that when fibroids have been absorbed through the process of autolysis they seldom recur, as is so often the case after surgical removal.

Fasting and the restriction of diet is best carried out under the supervision of a practitioner. He will be aware of the importance of the sparing diet being carefully balanced when it is designed to keep the weight at a level below normal. If this is not done there will be a distinct risk that malnutrition will result.

So little is known about nutrition that new discoveries are being made almost daily. This situation overwhelmingly supports the case for what we call the food reform regime and shows the fallacy of attempting to cure any serious ailment by prescribing single vital substances, whether they be mineral or vitamin, except in straightforward deficiency diseases like scurvy.

Synthetic vitamins are particularly liable to fail through lack of balance and this is why, unlike medical doctors, we naturopaths are always careful to prescribe vitamins known to be derived from natural sources. We are well aware that if we could be sure of obtaining a plentiful variety of unprocessed and uncontaminated food we should stand a chance of enjoying good health without the aid of supplementation, because such foods could be depended upon to contain all the micro-nutrients, both known and unknown, in the right proportion.

Since this is not the case, it is necessary to improvise as best we can. How then should the diet be worked out in the case of treating a fibroid tumour, so as to make provision on the one hand for weight reduction and on the other hand, for the correction of nutritional deficiencies which might be assumed to be a contributary cause of the malady?

The general requirements are a sufficiency of protein for the renewal of the cells of the body, but no more than that; enough carbohydrate to provide the body with energy, and all the vitamins, minerals and other micro-nutrients, some known and many unknown, in ample sufficiency and in the right propor-tions. This is what is achieved when we prescribe what has come to be called 'a balanced course of natural vitamins'.

Many of my women readers may be faced with the weighty decision whether they should obtain treatment for their fibroid tumour by conservative means, in the manner I have outlined, or submit to surgical removal. If, on discovery, the tumour is not large and does not give rise to pain or cause much inconvenience there would be a good case for relying upon natural therapy. At the other end of the scale would be a woman, not yet forty, with a fibroid equivalent to five months' pregnancy in outward appearance, giving rise to heavy men-strual loss and intermediate bleeding and causing pain both locally and through reflection to other organs. In this latter case surgical removal would seem to be a reasonable solution. It would be a great help in intermediate cases to have the advice of an unbiased naturopath with gynaecological experience in arriving at the right decision.

The nervous among you need not be afraid of being hurt, for we seldom use instruments in carrying out an examination. Experience enables a manual examination to discover all that is necessary.

Let me conclude this chapter with sensible advice. Do not submit to a gynaecological operation of any kind without first giving Nature Cure a chance to deal with the problem. The practitioner consulted, if he is suitably qualified, can be relied

upon to tell you frankly if your ailment is beyond his capacity
to treat.

## 18

## PROLAPSE OF THE UTERUS

Used as a medical term, 'prolapse' means the slipping down of some organ or structure. It can include a falling down of the intestines within the abdomen, when it is more precisely described as *visceroptosis*, or downward displacement of the bladder, the womb or the rectum. The latter disorder need only be mentioned briefly. It is a fairly frequent occurrence in children. Each time there is a bowel movement the lower end of the bowel protrudes outside the anus. When this happens it should be carefully sponged with cold water, replaced and, if necessary, retained in place with a soft pad and bandage attached to a waist belt.

*Visceroptosis* is a condition which may also begin early in life owing to weakness of the ligaments which support the abdominal organs and of the abdominal muscles. It is usually associated with faulty posture in standing. From the time they begin to walk and throughout their development parents are advised to carefully watch their children's posture when standing and encourage them to correct it when faulty. Not only will this attention prevent the appearance of the unsightly bulging tummy but also the hollow back, round shoulders and poking head all too common in today's youth. 'Deportment', as it used to be called in Victorian times, is just as important both for health reasons and aesthetically now as it always has been.

The prolapse which the gynaecologist is most often called upon to treat is that of the womb. When first seen, a prolapse of this kind may not be observable externally, even when the patient is standing. There is some discomfort and a 'bearing down' feeling but this is not severe. In the more pronounced forms of uterine prolapse the cervix will be found to project outside the vagina both when standing and when lying. Often it will be red and inflamed with chafing and there may be some bleeding. The patient sometimes wears a sanitary towel to afford protection and some support. Other cases have already been to a gynaecologist, who has fitted a supporting ring to be permanently worn within the vagina. The same gynaecologist may have explained that the wearing of a ring is no more than a temporary palliative and that the only effective solution would be to have a surgical operation performed. This would consist of manoeuvring the organ back into its normal position and then shortening the supporting ligaments or stitching it to adjoining tissue of the pelvic floor.

The treatment of uterine prolapse by surgery cannot be regarded as satisfactory because it does nothing to overcome the basic cause of the disorder, which is lack of tone in the womb itself, in the ligaments – whose purpose it is to hold it in its correct position – and in the soft tissue of the whole pelvic area. In severe cases surgery may be the only reasonable solution and if performed by a skilful surgeon will give a great deal of relief to the patient. In the event of the operation being inexpertly performed the patient's condition, thereafter, may be worse instead of better. It is the duty of the naturopathic practitioner to advise his patient if, in his opinion, the prolapse is too advanced to offer any hope of alleviation by the means at his disposal. In this event he would do his best to put his patient into contact with a surgeon likely to make a good job of the inevitable operation.

In explaining the procedure for treating a prolapse of the womb naturopathically and osteopathically, it must be pointed out that the general health of the patient is the first consideration. It would be futile to attempt treatment otherwise. We must make an assessment of the patient's nutritional condition and see to it that her diet is satisfactory. In most cases it will be necessary to prescribe supplementary nutrients because however carefully we choose the foods of today, many are less nutritious than we could wish. Also, we are up against the grave problem of pollution of the environment, which undermines our nutrition however good it may be and reduces our resistance to ill health. In prescribing supplementary nutrients, mostly vitamins, careful consideration must be given to quality and to the proper balance thereof. At the same time, should investigation disclose that there is a marked deficiency in one particular vitamin, more of this should be included in the course.

### Inadequate Circulation
Provision having been made for the nutritional integrity of the patient, the next consideration must be the circulation – remembering the all-important role of the blood in keeping the

organs in a healthy condition. Many ailments to which the flesh is heir result from inadequate circulation and the reason for this can easily be made clear. The chief function of the blood is the renewal of cells, of which every part of the body is formed. In every organ literally millions of cells wear out every day and they have to be taken away and replaced by new cells. It is not difficult to understand that if this function is not efficiently performed, ill health in organs will be manifested by malfunction and by the growth of cysts and tumours, and in the joints and muscles by rheumatism and arthritis when the accumulation of toxic matter becomes chronic, or by transient aches and pains which are intended to act as a warning signal that all is not well with the circulation.

One of the results of inadequate circulation is lack of tone in the muscles and ligaments whose function is to support the organs, and this – of course – applies to the womb and also to the bladder and the rectum which adjoin it.

Since the motive power for circulation is provided by the heart, we must see to it that this organ is in good shape and if it is not prescribe suitable herbal remedies to improve its function.

A form of light osteopathy, which we call neuromuscular manipulation, is always given when the circulation is known to be inadequate and is very beneficial, not only for this reason but also in stimulating the nervous system which controls the working of all organs.

Exercises are taught for two reasons, firstly, to improve the breathing capacity and thereby the oxygenation of the blood and, secondly, for the purpose of gaining conscious control of the pelvic organs, but more of this later.

### Correcting a Prolapsed Womb

Osteopathic gynaecology properly applied can work wonders in correcting a prolapsed womb. Readers who have reason for concern about the malady will be interested to hear something of the technique employed.

After the patient has emptied the bladder and rectum she is placed in the knee-chest position. This allows the intestines to gravitate away from the pelvis, and thus congestion is relieved. The cervix is now pressed firmly, but gently, in the direction of the pelvic cavity. The pressure must be steady but not hurried. After replacement, a sweeping movement, commencing first in the front of the womb and then on each side is given. This depletes the congested vaginal walls as well as the tissues between the layers of ligaments supporting the womb. The patient is instructed to assume the knee-chest position for several minutes before retiring at night and after carrying out the special pelvic exercises briefly referred to above.

The purpose of these exercises is to enable the patient to gain conscious control of the uterine ligaments and of the musclature in the whole pelvic area. This is not a normal ability but it can be acquired by concentration of the mind on the parts involved. The practitioner will be able to note progress in this direction each time he gives internal treatment.

In the more serious cases, at the commencement of treatment the cervix will be found to project outside the vagina, resulting in much soreness. To allay this the best remedy is a herbal ointment derived from the humble chickweed. This is very soothing and has great healing properties.

Remedies that work from within in helping to restore circulation and the tone of the affected parts must not be overlooked. These can be both herbal and homoeopathic. Examples are *Aletris Farinosa* (unicorn root), *China Regia* (smilax), *Helonias Dioica* (starwort), *Pulsatilla* (anemone pulsatilla) and *Lilium Tigrinum* (tiger lily).

In closing I think a word of advice should be given to younger women who are not afflicted with the distressing disorder which has been described. Most of these cases could have been avoided altogether by early precautions. There is much to be said for having a gynaecological check-up when the forties are reached. The examination might disclose a less serious displacement of the womb or a general lack of tone which could subsequently worsen and give a great deal of trouble. Suitable treatment at this stage would give far more speedy results than would be the case if nothing is done until a prolapse has become obvious.

### Sensational Items

In the space remaining it may be helpful to comment on the sensational items concerning the welfare of women that appear in the newspapers and in radio and TV programmes with great frequency. It is appreciated that the publicity media must always be on the look out for news items and the more sensational they are the better, from the point of view of capturing the interest of the public. The complaint I would make about all this is that there is hardly ever any balanced comment on these sensational news items, with the result that women are often left with a feeling of puzzlement and bewilderment.

In April 1970 there was a report in *The Times* of a talk by Professor Jeffcoate, President of the Royal College of Obstetricians and Gynaecologists, at the European Congress of Prenatal Medicine held in London.

First the Professor pointed out that in considering the care of the baby before birth, the foetus within the mother's womb is no longer regarded as a massive parasite but as an individual whose alimentary, renal, metabolic, endocrine and nervous system contributed to the whole complex. It even controlled its own development in many respects and might determine its birthday.

Speculating on future possibilities, Professor Jeffcoate said that if a baby drank before birth as it did after birth, why not devise something comparable to milk, or at least a bland concentrate of high nutritional value, which could be injected daily for the foetus to absorb?

It would seem that no attempt was made by the Professor or anyone else to explain that this procedure, which must sound horrifying to many women, would only be justified in cases where the mother-to-be is so seriously ill that the welfare of her baby is in jeopardy because she can no longer adequately nourish it. Unfortunately for those of us who have to finance the National Health Service with the taxes we pay, the medical profession are for ever on the lookout for methods which are elaborate and costly — both in time and in money — whilst they abandon the simple, and often more successful, procedures of the past. Many a disgusted patient has come to me in desperation for help after spending two or three days in hospital, during which time she has had to endure the whole gamut of elaborate diagnostic procedures with instruments and chemicals only to face the anti-climax of being told that nothing wrong could be found. For many it was a sad day when doctors ceased to be trained to use their hands and their eyes and their ears to aid their diagnosis, as they did in the past so successfully.

In the case of the mother-to-be, I have constantly urged that her nutrition must be the chief concern of the practitioner who takes care of her. In the vast majority of cases this will do more than anything to ensure that her baby will be healthy and contented from birth onwards, whilst she, herself, will come through the ordeal with the minimum of distress. This is how nature intended it to be and I am sure nature would abhor the idea of injecting nutrients into the unborn child whilst still within its mother's womb. To the unsophisticated among us it sounds too much like taking a sledge-hammer to crack a nut.

More recently we listened to a woman doctor who quite calmly, via the radio, informed us that she had 'prescribed' the birth pill for her two-year-old daughter about a dozen times in the last year. This was done, she said, to demonstrate to women that the pill is not dangerous. It does not speak well for medical education that the doctor in question must have been oblivious of the fact that the long-term effect on women of taking the pill will not be known for a further twenty years or more. This we are told on the authority of scientists, whose business it is to rigorously screen all new drugs before their administration by doctors is permitted. The pills which the doctor in question gave to her baby daughter so light-heartedly contained powerful synthetic hormones which are known to be capable of having very serious long-term effects on the well-being of adult women who take them. Surely they could have still more disastrous effects on the developing organs of a baby girl. Unfortunately, this radio talk was not followed by any authoritative comment which would have served to preserve the balance in the minds of listeners. I think it should have been.

## 19

## BREAST DISORDERS:
## AVOIDING MALIGNANCY

Women should be encouraged to examine their breasts periodically as a matter of routine. Once a month at mid-period in women who have not reached the menopause is suggested, and a similar interval in older women. This advice will not lead to 'cancerphobia' if a sensible attitude is cultivated. A woman's familiarity with the normal feel and texture of her breasts assists her to recognize any changes that may occur. The most common change is by no means an ominous one suggesting cancer but that which is brought about by the growth of simple cysts. For every woman who contracts a breast cancer at least ten will discover one or more of these cysts.

A cyst is a sac or capsule containing fluid or fibre, but mostly the former. When first located they may be smaller than a pea but they are liable to slowly increase in size and may not be discovered until they are as large as a walnut for cysts are usually quite painless. A characteristic of breast cysts is that they appear to be 'floating' in the breast tissue and are thus freely movable.

When a woman discovers that she has a 'lump' in the breast she should not conclude that it is just a cyst and think no more about it. She should make an appointment to see her doctor or practitioner so that its true nature can be determined.

Should professional examination disclose that the lump has the characteristics of a tumour and not those of a cyst, it by no means follows that the tumour is a malignant one. A considerable proportion of breast tumours are benign when first discovered.

Indications other than a lump which should be properly investigated are:

Any alteration in the shape of the breast.
Elevation or sinking of the nipple.
Slight dimpling of the skin of the breast.
Discharge, bleeding or rash around the nipple.

Early breast cancer is almost always painless and for this reason the victim is liable to remark, 'Oh yes, I've noticed a lump there for months but it hasn't bothered me at all.' Pain is not an early warning signal.

## Mastitis

Pain in the breast is usually associated with mastitis, which is a different disorder. It is not due to infection, but to some disturbance of the hormone balance. It occurs with increasing frequency after the age of thirty years and is more common in women who have borne children. The pain is usually worse just before the onset of a monthly period. It may be confined to one part of the breast or it may involve the whole breast or both breasts. There may be some swelling and a feeling of heaviness. The condition may be worsened by allowing the mind to dwell upon it and by constant handling. It is important that a well-fitting brassière giving adequate support from underneath be worn. Fortunately, medical herbalists have remedies which usually bring early relief in simple cases. I have found the best of these to be one called *Conium*. This is derived from Indian hemp, otherwise known as cannabis or hashish. Readers will recognize it as one of the prohibited drugs but we use it in a homoeopathic potency, which is in no way harmful and quite permissible.

In cases of mastitis which are resistant to this promising treatment, hormone imbalance is likely to be responsible. Herbal remedies which have the capacity of encouraging the body to produce its own hormones in the right proportion are then administered.

Acute inflammation and abscess formation is liable to occur when breast-feeding a baby. The infection usually reaches the breast from the nipple as a result of cracks in it and lack of cleanliness. It can also result from an indrawn or sunken nipple.

This is a case where prevention should receive full consideration. For several weeks before delivery a pregnant woman should carefully massage her nipples daily using *Chickweed* ointment as a lubricant. This will keep the nipples soft and healthy. If the baby is — as one would hope — breast-fed, scrupulous attention to cleansing the breast and nipples must be observed each time the baby is put to the breast, by sponging with warm water which has been boiled, followed by gentle massaging using *Chickweed* ointment as a lubricant. Should ulceration threaten either before or after delivery, development can often be arrested by suitable treatment. A homoeopathic practitioner would probably prescribe *Bryonia Alba 3* or *Phytolacca 1* and apply a hot fomentation of *Calendula* lotion to the affected area at frequent intervals. If in spite of these precautions an abscess develops, it might have to be opened and drained.

In a case in which a non-medical practitioner, on examining his patient, is left in no doubt that the swelling is of a suspicious nature, he should refer her to a physician or surgeon for a second opinion. Should this second examination confirm the likelihood of malignancy the patient would be recommended to submit to surgery immediately.

If there is no more than a nucleus of malignancy it is liable to spread rapidly to adjoining areas, including the lymph nodes under the arm pit. Surgical removal is then fraught with the risk of what is known as 'metastasis', meaning the invasion of other parts of the body by cancer cells set free by the operation. At the commencement of an operation it is usual for a microscopic examination of a small piece of the tissue (called a 'biopsy') to be made. If this indicates that the tumour is benign (non-malignant) this alone need be removed and the breast itself left intact with little or no disfigurement.

Understandably, women are apt to regard removal of a breast as a serious disfigurement and resent the operation for this reason. There is some compensation in the fact that the disfigurement can be rectified by the wearing of a surgical breast form, and these are readily available.

Following the operation, most surgeons will advise treatment of the chest area with X-rays, the purpose of which is to destroy any stray malignant cells that might have been missed through being too deep-seated.

## Not a Death Sentence

The medical profession claims that it is a fallacy to suppose breast malignancy constitutes a death sentence. It is said, on the contrary, that more than 65 per cent of women who have had a diseased breast removed are living active and useful lives years afterwards. It is pointed out that we always hear of the patient who does not do well after the operation, but the thousands every year whose lives are unchanged or improved by mastectomy do not hit the headlines.

A serious failing for which we of the unorthodox fraternity feel obliged to criticize the medical profession is that, excepting on rare occasions, nothing is done prior to a surgical operation to build up the patient's ability to come through the ordeal with a minimum of distress and make a quick recovery from the shock afterwards.

We can offer substantial help in this direction if called upon to do so. Commencing at least a month before the operation is to be performed, the patient should be advised about her diet — which should be wholesome and nourishing. Maximum nutrition should be ensured by prescribing, in addition, a balanced course of natural vitamins with special emphasis in this case on vitamin C. We now have substantial evidence that the presence of this vitamin in the system in generous quantity will expedite the healing process. On the other hand it has not been found, so far, that comparatively massive doses of up to two or three grams a day have been in any way harmful. Should there be a surplus above the needs of the body it will be freely eliminated.

Other grounds upon which there must be criticism is that the large sums of money publicly prescribed to defeat the menace of cancer are almost exclusively in support of research on finding a *cure* for cancer. In my view and that of many others of like persuasion, there should be far more emphasis on *seeking the cause* of cancer and the prevention thereof.

There can be little doubt that the very serious pollution of the whole of our environment, which has become such a problem, has much to do with the steady increase we are witnessing, not only in cancer of various kinds but other chronic degenerative diseases as well. There is reason for gratification that both the public and those in authority are at last becoming aware of the grave menace to health that this pollution problem presents.

**Rules for Wholesome Living**

Many forms of pollution, of which that of motor vehicle exhausts is an example, cannot be avoided by the individual but the individual can do a good deal to combat pollution by building up his (or her) resistance to it by trying to live wholesomely. Here are suggestions to this end.

1. A lacto-vegetarian diet should be adopted as closely as convenient and every effort be made to obtain food from sources that have not been contaminated with chemicals.

2. Within reason, avoid foods that have been tinned and packaged, especially if they have at the same time been excessively processed, over-refined, and otherwise denatured. The over-cooking of foods is also likely to be harmful.

3. Although the difficulties may be insuperable for some, every effort should be made to obtain organically grown foods. Those who have gardens should most certainly aim at producing as much as possible of their own fruit and vegetable supplies using organic methods.

4. A virtually salt-free diet should be adopted, whilst foods having a high potassium content should be favoured. Among these foods are:

| | |
|---|---|
| Apples | Salads of all kinds. |
| Bananas | Carrots |
| Grapes | Potatoes (preferably cooked in jackets). |
| Citrus fruits | Tomatoes |
| All green vegetables | Dried peas and lentils and the many kinds of bean. |
| Oats in any form. | |

In adhering to a salt-free diet it must be borne in mind that many tinned, packaged, and processed foods are likely to have a comparatively high salt content.

5. Aluminium cooking utensils and pressure cookers should not be used. In pressure cookers the high temperature produced is destructive of vitamins.

6. Smoking should be given up and stimulating beverages such as tea, coffeee and cocoa reduced to a minimum. It is possible to obtain decaffeinated coffee and coffee substitutes that do not contain caffein in health food shops. For those who would regard it as a hardship to give up tea altogether it is recommended that one cup of tea of the highest quality and affording the maximum of enjoyment be drunk where three cups of ordinary tea were drunk previously. Although the high quality tea would cost more there would still be an overall saving. Various herbal teas and drinks made from fresh fruit juices or vegetable juices are all excellent substitutes for the more common but over-stimulating and non-nutritious beverages. *Chamomile* tea is highly recommended.

7. Those unwilling to adhere strictly to a vegetarian diet can have fish occasionally in preference to meat but it must be fresh. If there is a preference for chicken or other poultry, those which have been produced by the broiler or some other intensive system should be ruled out. Poultry reared on free range and eggs from the same source are altogether better.

8. All forms of animal fat and hydrogenated oils and fats

must be excluded from the diet. This prohibition will include most margarine and cooking fats but there are now margarines on the market that have not been subject to excessive hydro-generation. Vegetable oils, especially sunflower seed and corn oil, may be used freely, both raw with salads and in cooking where oil or fat is needed. All are available in health food shops. As a special treat unsalted butter may be used occasionally by those who are very fond of butter. Cheese may be used fairly liberally. Cottage cheese and the less sophisticated varieties of hard cheese such as *Cheddar* are preferable.

9. White sugar and confectionery made with white sugar, and beverages in which white sugar and saccharine are used, should be excluded from the diet and unrefined sugar, such as barbados and demerara, be insisted upon. Honey may be eaten freely provided the subject is not overweight.

10. Other items best avoided are frozen foods, bottled drinks which cannot be guaranteed free, or virtually free, from chemical additives; baking powder and soda, epsom and other purgative salts; liquid paraffin; white flour; ice cream; (but dairy ice cream is preferable to the synthetic varieties); hair dyes and many cosmetics including the hormonized products. As regards baking powder, it is appreciated that the traditional variety made with carbonate of soda and tartaric acid has been used for generations. Provided no chemicals other than these are included in one's baking powder, and neither it nor carbonate of soda by itself are used excessively, they are unlikely to be harmful.

11. The breathing capacity should be improved by learning to carry out simple breathing exercises. The average person only uses one-third of his lung capacity. Inefficient breathing deprives the cells of the body of an adequate oxygen supply and this can lead to cell deterioration, which is a precursor of cancer.

12. Cancer cases are often preceded by a long history of constipation. It is most important that obstinate constipation be corrected by natural means, mainly through the diet. If laxatives are indispensable at first, they must be herbal preparations.

13. All the available evidence goes to show that overweight is inimical to good health. By rigorously controlling diet, normal weight must be maintained. Weight reduction by means of drugs can be extremely dangerous. In a restricted diet care must be

taken to preserve a balance so that an adequate supply of foods containing minerals and vitamins is retained.

14. Owing to the extreme difficulty in getting an adequate supply of foods that have been grown in truly fertile soil and have not been contaminated by chemicals and excessively processed, the use of nutritional supplements has become almost essential. These should consist of products derived exclusively from natural sources, such as brewer's yeast for vitamin B-complex, and rose hip capsules for vitamin C. Artificial vitamin products synthetically produced should be avoided. It is important to preserve a proper balance when taking supplementary nutrients and not take an excess of one vital substance and exclude others. If in doubt about this point it would be wise to consult a practitioner knowledgeable about food reform nutrition. In the long run considerable economy could be effected through obtaining expert advice.

## 20

# THE MENOPAUSE

Many books and innumerable articles have been written on the health problem with which every woman is confronted as she approaches middle age. In familiar language we call it 'the change'. I make no apology for embarking upon yet another review of this important subject, as seen from a naturopathic angle. As in all other aspects of the healing art, the means at our disposal for ameliorating human suffering in this sphere become greater with the passage of time although our basic principles remain the same.

In spite of all that has been written there remains a great deal of misunderstanding among women about the menopause, including the age of its onset.

The Ancient Greeks called the menopause the climacteric, meaning the step of a ladder. They supposed the whole body was renewed every seven years and looked upon some of these periods as of special importance. There is some justification for this view. At fourteen the average girl reaches puberty and sexual activity appears in the shape of menstruation. At about twenty-one we consider that full sexual maturity has been attained, rendering this the most appropriate age for marriage. At forty-two, or thereabouts, we are accustomed to expect that menstruation and the capacity to bear children will cease.

Actually, the age at which the onset of menopause occurs in the majority of women is between their forty-sixth and fiftieth years. Women who begin to menstruate early in life usually have a long menstrual record and a late menopause. However, this is far from a constant rule. In my experience it is rare for the change to begin before the age of forty-five but many women have attended me when well on in the fifties, who were still menstruating.

## Menstruation: Nature's Marvel

The physiological processes related to the menstruation of women is one of the marvels of nature and must be briefly described as a prelude to explaining the manner of its ending.

The normal female child is born with two ovaries, each one

of which contains a fixed number of ova; ova being the minute eggs from which a new life can begin. When a girl reaches the appropriate stage of development an ovum breaks out of one of her ovaries and approximately fourteen days later she will menstruate for the first time.

The ovum emerges from the ovary in a capsule or follicle which bursts and releases it when it is free to find its way into the womb. Also released is a substance called the *corpus luteum*. This in turn, aided by stimulus from the pituitary gland, produces the hormones progesterone and oestrogen, which enter the blood stream. If fertilization of the ovum does not occur, the corpus luteum, after functioning for about twelve days, begins to degenerate and ceases to secrete progesterone. The effect of the absence of progesterone, together with a diminution in the amount of oestrogen in the blood, renders the lining of the womb unstable so that this breaks away about fourteen days after ovulation with resulting haemorrhage and a new menstrual flow begins.

If no fertilization of the ovum, released each month from the ovary, occurs as a result of sexual intercourse, the process of discharge and renewal of the lining of the womb every twenty-eight days on average will regularly continue throughout the life of a healthy woman from puberty until the last of the ova which her ovaries originally contained has been discharged. The story of conception, pregnancy and childbirth is also a miraculous one, but does not belong here.

It has now been made clear that the symptoms of ill-health associated with the menopause are due, in the main, to failure of the ovaries to produce the oestrogenic hormones associated with them when all the ova have been used up. Before describing the treatment which is available to make good the deficiency, I will relate some of the changes and disorders from which women are liable to suffer at that time. To some extent her femininity is diminished since the hormone (now deficient) contributes to the softness of her skin, the shapeliness of her body and to sexual lubrication. Some women, though by no means all, approach the neuter stage after the menopause with a deepened voice, coarser complexion and an increase in facial hair. By far the most common and distressing menopausal disorder is the occurrence of hot flushes, sometimes accompanied by excessive perspiration and perhaps feelings of faintness. This particular symptom is worthy of note by the practitioner because it gives a useful indication of the hormone level of the subject. Not all women have hot flushes at the time of the menopause; flushes do not commonly precede it and may not begin until some years after the actual cessation of menstruation.

## Melancholia

In the mental sphere the commonest and most characteristic indication is melancholia. This is in part a direct consequence of hormonal withdrawal, although the fact that the mood is lowered makes one look for – and usually find – sad aspects in the patient's life at that time. A woman often feels sad and depressed because the menopause marks the end of an era. No longer is she capable of bearing children and her youth and beauty will fade henceforth. Her children have grown up and left the fold. She has become very dependent for companionship on her husband and a lot depends upon the warmth of the marital relationship that has been maintained.

It is customary for medical doctors when treating such deficiency symptoms as hot flushes and melancholia to embark upon what is known as substitution therapy. They prescribe replacement dosages of oestrogen. We naturopaths disagree with this form of treatment for several reasons. Firstly the weapon is a two-edged one and the side-effects can be worse than the ailment for which it is prescribed. The hormones used are usually synthetic and it is admitted that there is a great deal still to learn about their use, even when, as is sometimes the case, a hormone derived from animal sources is administered. Doctors acknowledge too that there are chemical reasons for hazarding, and clinical reasons for supposing that oestrogens, especially synthetic ones, have some connection with the onset of cancer.

The implications and risks of hormone therapy have become much greater with the advent of the contraceptive pill, which itself consists of synthetic hormones. It will be many years before the full effect on the gynaecological health of women of saturating them with these chemicals will be known but it could be just as disastrous as the misuse of antibiotics has now proved to be. I particularly deplore the light-hearted way in which the pill is now being made available for young girls. How wrong it is that the risk should be taken of permanently deranging those most intricate and delicate organs and processes of reproduction when they have only just begun to function. We might well weep for our folly. However, in wholeheartedly and un-reservedly condemning the employment of synthetic hormones in the treatment of the menopause I am far from suggesting that we should do nothing and just allow nature to run its course.

## A Complete Check-Up

First of all I advocate most strongly that all women, whatever the strength of their belief in Nature Cure may be, should at the age of forty seek a consultation with a practitioner experienced in gynaecology with a view to having a complete check-up of their general and gynaecological health. When seeking an appointment they should make it clear that this is what they require and obtain confirmation that it will be carried out.

Never have we had a better example of the importance of the 'stitch in time' than we have here. Years of misery can often be saved by the right form of treatment at this stage. Aches, pains, lumps, bumps, shows (vaginal discharge), haemorrhages, weight gain or loss, indigestion, depression; everything that might take a woman to a practitioner at another time of life should certainly do so at the age of forty or thereabouts.

If as a result of his examination the practitioner in his role of gynaecologist, does not find any obvious pathological disorder such as fibroid, ovarian cyst, inflammation of the womb, polyps or erosion of the cervix, all of which have to be specially treated, his assistance will take the form of making sure that the patient's way of life is in keeping with the situation. Is her dieting all that it should be? Is her background a happy one?

If I were attending a woman who at the age of forty or thereabouts had come to see me for a check-up I should first of all satisfy myself that there was nothing amiss in the organs with which I am chiefly concerned, those of reproduction. If this had not already been done I should recommend the carrying out of the cervical smear test so as to exclude the possibility of there being anything suspicious in the condition of the cervix beyond that which the straightforward gynae-cological examination will disclose. This test I should prefer to carry out myself because when it is done through National Health provisions it is usually impossible to get an accurate assessment of the condition if the report is anything but negative.

Few women appreciate that there are many degrees of involvement short of liability to cancer when the report is not a negative one, and most of these can be conservatively treated at the right time.

Also requiring special attention would be the condition of the outer part of the vagina, which at the age of forty in some women begins to lose its elasticity, thus rendering intercourse uncomfortable if not intolerable. This is a danger signal demanding immediate treatment because a few years later it could render normal marital relations impossible.

## Nutritional Status

We must now ask ourselves the question; why is it that some women go through the critical years of the menopause with no unpleasant symptoms at all whilst others have the lot? In my view the answer lies primarily in the nutritional status of the subject. The body is short of the basic vital substances needed for the adequate supply of essential hormones and for the stimulation of the glands responsible for hormone production. The treatment I shall prescribe will aim at making sure before it is too late that there will not be this fatal dearth of hormone-producing substances at the time when they are most urgently needed.

As in all cases, the patient's dietary regime must be closely questioned and if this is not all that it should be she is urged to reform and is provided with instructions to this end. She will also be advised to carry out some simple exercises designed to improve the circulation and increase her breathing capacity.

A well-ordered diet may not alone ensure that all the essential vital substances will be available. As we grow older our need for these becomes greater whilst we may have to make up for years of partial deprivation. We have to give supplementary nutrients, otherwise vitamins and minerals. These must be derived from natural sources, for we can have no confidence in synthetic vitamins.

The chemical similarity of some of the vitamins to some of the hormones has been well established by research and in particular by Dr M.S. Biskind. Biochemists not only agree that vitamins can replace hormones in certain circumstances but point out that when taken by mouth are molecularly capable of being absorbed through the small intestine into the blood stream with greater facility than are the hormones themselves.

The two hormones with which we are particularly concerned are oestrogen and progesterone. In substitution therapy we need

Vitamin A for the former and Vitamin C for the latter. Research workers in this field freely acknowledge the complexity of the subject and it is not yet clear how the body performs its miracles of converting one vital substance into another but we do know that the pituitary gland (sometimes referred to as the master gland) plays an important part in directing these intricate processes. It is also believed that Vitamin E reserves not only permit a more efficient utilization of other vitamins and Vitamin A in particular, but exercises an important influence over the overall function of the pituitary gland.

### Herbal Treatment

Still more recent research in Germany and Sweden has proved beyond doubt that extracts from the herb *Agnus Castus* used medicinally exercise an activating effect upon *corpus luteum* and hormone production through the pituitary gland. *Agnus Castus* is a shrub indigenous in countries bordering the Mediterranean and has a history going back to antiquity as a sovereign remedy for disorders of the female genital organs.

Herbs which contain a natural form of oestrogen may also be prescribed to serve as a temporary bridge whilst the body is making adjustment to suit the situation. Among these are the familiar liquorice and the less familiar unicorn roots. One has the Latin name *Aletris Farinosa* and the other *Chamaelirium Luteum*.

We now have a fairly clear picture of how to proceed if we wish to alleviate the severity of the menopause. In my experience I have found that it is not good therapy to give the significant vitamins A and C alone but as part of a balanced course of vitamins. It has to be borne in mind that deprivation symptoms are liable to persist if a lot of one vitamin is prescribed and others are ignored. The herbal remedy may be administered alone or in combination with other herbal remedies, depending on the general picture. Not infrequently the menopause is accompanied by one or more other disorders which are brought to light at the time of the examination and these, of course, must also be treated.

The essence of the advice that this chapter brings to women of forty or thereabouts is that however well you may be feeling, now is the time to seek an appointment with a practitioner who will give you a careful check-up, not only of your physical condition but also of your mode of living and will then advise what changes could be made with advantage. He will make sure that you are getting all the vitamins you need to keep you fit and healthy and well able to stand up successfully to the menopause when it comes, and prescribe suitable treatment in the event of some unsuspected disorder being brought to light.

## 21

# 'THE PILL': WHAT ARE THE RISKS?

Both my private misgivings and responsibility to my readers makes it imperative that I should once again take upon myself the task of protesting against the uncritical acceptance of the contraceptive pill.

In our newspapers and magazines it has become the custom, whenever the question of contraception is discussed, to almost always take it for granted that contraception and 'the pill' are virtually synonymous terms.

Unfortunately, terminology is, in considerable measure, responsible for what has happened. It is so much easier for journalists to use a slick term such as 'the pill', which even children have now come to recognize instantly, than the cumbersome descriptions of the older, much less hazardous forms of contraception.

This development, initially fortuitous, and subsequently fostered by subtle propaganda, must be a source of immense satisfaction to pharmaceutical manufacturers. It has accelerated immeasurably what is probably the greatest windfall this industry ever had.

With practically no effort, and little expense in advertising, the pill has quickly become one of the best sellers among pharmaceutical products. Doctors, most of whom are grossly overworked, are also known to bless the pill as one of the most effective time-savers that has ever come their way.

Women who visit my consulting room for the conservative treatment afforded them by naturopathy, keep me very well informed. No longer does the average doctor bother to delve into the intricacies of hormone therapy, when confronted with a variety of gynaecological problems. The pill provides him with blended hormones ready for use.

If your daughter, having reached the age of fifteen, has failed to menstruate, the pill will be prescribed to make her do so. If you have painful menstrual disorder, the pill will once again be offered. Most incongruous of all is the fact that the pill is frequently prescribed in cases of infertility!

To better illustrate the way in which the use of the pill by women is now taken for granted, let me mention a single incident.

Only yesterday a mother told me her daughter, aged nineteen, was about to be married. On going to the family doctor for some pre-marital advice, he remarked that she seemed to be the kind of girl who would easily conceive. 'I had better provide you with the pill,' said he. I am glad to say her family background was such that she had the good sense to refuse the offer.

Publicity for the pill increased greatly in volume when it was thought that because of the rebellious attitude of many of its members, the Roman Catholic Church might look more favourably on contraception in general. One saw headlines such as, 'Will Catholics Accept the Pill?'

Publicity rose to even greater heights when Malcolm Muggeridge resigned the Rectorship of Edinburgh University because he did not think it right that promiscuity among students should be encouraged by making contraception too freely available. For several days television, radio and the press gave the matter top priority. Always, speakers and journalists made it appear that the pill and contraception meant the same thing.

The Muggeridge versus university students episode will have done incalculable harm, by making it appear to young girls that contraception and the pill are synonymous terms. Added to this is the fact that there are hardly any complexities in using the pill. All the girl has to do for her safety is to take the pill for twenty days of her menstrual cycle.

For easy use the pills are put up in a dispenser holding the correct number, and the day on which dosage should commence is clearly indicated. The pill is omitted during eight days of the cycle so that menstruation will be permitted to occur.

### Health Menace

The stage has now been set for me to explain why taking the pill must be regarded as a menace to the health of women. It has been in use for several years and it is estimated that in the U.S.A. alone, for twenty days every month, 6½ million women — one out of every five in the childbearing years — now take this birth-control remedy. The ease and effectiveness of the method has revolutionized contraception.

At the same time, the pill has created an unprecedented

dilemma for conscientious doctors and patients. In the history of medicine, no other drug has been so widely prescribed for a purpose not directly related to the treatment of disease. Yet there is still no clear-cut verdict on its safety.

Reports coming in from doctors and women regarding the pill have been so alarming that the leading authority on family planning in the U.S.A., the American College of Obstetricians and Gynaecologists, with a fellowship of 7,000, decided that the time had come to carry out an exhaustive survey in which all its fellows would participate.

The purpose of the survey was to reveal exactly what are the risks, as well as the benefits, of oral contraceptives.

Although the effectiveness and convenience of the pill were fully established by this vast survey, it also became abundantly clear there are so many hazards that the remedy must not be considered a harmless drug to be dispensed casually.

Women using the pill must be kept under constant observation by their physician and note taken of physical and emotional symptoms that the ovulation-suppressing hormones of the pill are liable to induce. Some doctors commented, in the margin of their report, 'I prescribe, but do not recommend the pill'.

A complete review of this most valuable investigation has been prepared by Alice Lake and was published in McCalls magazine of November 1967. I am indebted to one of my patients, a young girl, for not only drawing my attention to the report, but kindly presenting me with her copy of McCalls. Although more than six years have passed since the report was published, during which time attempts have been made to modify it, the basic objections to it have not diminished.

## When the Pill is Dangerous

Limitations of space will only permit me to give you a brief summary. For women who have problems with varicose veins, phlebitis and blood clotting, and women who are liable to contract cancer, the pill would be quite definitely harmful. These latter include patients who have had breast tumours, or benign cysts of the breast, and those who have a family history of cancer. The pill will also harm women who suffer from water-retention with liability to swollen ankles. These include cases of heart diseases, asthma and epilepsy.

Women with liver disorders are bad subjects for the pill. This is because the liver is the organ which breaks down the estrogen (a component of the pill). With the organ functioning normally, excessive amounts of the hormone would circulate in the bloodstream with damaging results.

In women who have a proneness to jaundice, severe itching, brownish facial spots and deep depression the pill may be expected to aggravate the symptoms.

Women who are potential diabetics should not take the pill. They belong in this category if they have had adverse results in blood-sugar tests, or if close members of the family have diabetes. Also in this category are women who have delivered unusually large babies.

The pill should be rejected by women who get migraine headaches, especially if the headaches worsen soon after the pill has been tried.

Perhaps the most important of all cases where the pill would be prohibited by most of the gynaecologists participating in the investigation, are women of potential limited fertility. Those who have a history of irregular or scanty menstruation fall into this category. It is considered that pill-taking would reduce their chances of pregnancy when this was desired at a chosen time.

Among the more general symptoms which ought to be considered a reason for avoiding the pill are severe headaches, bleeding between periods, jaundice, unusually dark urine, pain or tenderness in the calf of the leg, liability to chest pain, difficulty in keeping weight under control and – please take note – women who have fibroid tumours of the uterus which are small and trouble-free and do not warrant surgical removal.

More than half the specialists taking part in the survey were convinced that the pill quickened the growth of fibroids.

Setting aside this monumental investigation, which clearly shows that there are innumerable cases in which taking the pill would be detrimental to a woman's health, let us look at another aspect of the problem.

### American Doctor's Condemnation

Dr David Klebanow, M.D., a senior gynaecologist in Mount Sinai Hospital, New York, severely condemns the use of the pill in a monologue published in 1963. He first draws attention to the bitter fight the medical world witnessed forty years ago concerning the use of X-ray radiation to bring about temporary cessation of menstruation in gynaecological conditions such as excessive menstrual bleeding and inflammation of the womb.

This therapeutic procedure was accepted and practised by the medical profession throughout the world, until research workers in France and the U.S.A. raised the question of possible damage to unfertilized eggs, with adverse effect upon the products of conception when ovulation and subsequent pregnancies started to recur.

After several years of argument, accepted and rejected experiments on laboratory animals, and data from patients, in 1927 it was finally proved beyond doubt that this X-ray therapy could cause degenerative changes in the ova within the ovaries. This brought about an end to this form of X-ray radiation therapy.

Increase in knowledge over the years has confirmed that not only are eggs (ova) damaged, but the chromosomes within them are also affected. Considering that the chromosomes determine what kind of off-spring a woman will bear, the adverse effect on posterity of X-rays is all too obvious.

Doctor Klebanow has grave doubts as to the wisdom of administering hormones in the form of the contraceptive pill. There is sufficient evidence that these steroids can have a similarly damaging effect on the ovarian follicular apparatus, and the ova which they contain, that X-rays would have, and that the safety of future generations could be jeopardized.

He suggests that the use of the pill could give rise to malformations, especially mongoloids.

It is an accepted principle that substances that aggravate existing ailments can also initiate or cause a proneness to the same ailments. Thus we are faced with the shocking prospect of young girls, who have only recently become capable of bearing children, having the most wonderful and delicately balanced apparatus with which nature has endowed them – the reproductive system – thrown out of gear at the very outset of their womanhood.

I implore parents who have some influence over their daughters to beg them to think twice before accepting this form of contraception, with all its possibilities of permanent damage to their health and reproductive capacity, to say nothing of the possible menace to the children they may one day bear.

In giving this advice I am not unmindful that recourse to contraception is altogether preferable to procuring an abortion but the older, reasonably effective, and virtually harmless methods of contraception are still available.

# INDEX

IRWIN SHAW.

Sailor off the Bremen.
The young Lions
The Troubled Air
Mixed Company.
Lucy Crown.
Tip on a dead jockey
Two weeks in another town.
Rich man, Poor man. ✓